D1165661

SHAKEN BRAIN

SHAKEN BRAIN

The **SCIENCE, CARE,** and **TREATMENT** of **CONCUSSION**

Elizabeth Sandel, MD

Harvard University Press

Cambridge, Massachusetts
London, England
2020

First printing

Many of the designations used by manufacturers and sellers to distinguish their
products are claimed as trademarks. Where those designations appear in this book
and Harvard University Press was aware of a trademark claim, then the designations
have been printed in initial capital letters.

Library of Congress Cataloging-in-Publication Data
Names: Sandel, Elizabeth, author.
Title: Shaken brain : the science, care, and treatment of concussion /
    Elizabeth Sandel, MD.
Description: Cambridge, Massachusetts : Harvard University Press, 2020. |
    Includes bibliographical references and index.
Identifiers: LCCN 2019040007 (print) | LCCN 2019040008 (ebook) |
    ISBN 9780674987418 (cloth) | ISBN 9780674246324 (adobe pdf) |
    ISBN 9780674246331 (epub) | ISBN 9780674246348 (mobi)
Subjects: LCSH: Brain—Concussion. | Brain damage—Treatment. |
    Sports injuries.
Classification: LCC RC394.C7 S26 2020 (print) | LCC RC394.C7 (ebook) |
    DDC 616.8—dc23
LC record available at https://lccn.loc.gov/2019040007
LC ebook record available at https://lccn.loc.gov/2019040008

In memory of my parents, George and Kay Sandel,

for giving me a love of language, learning, and teaching

AND

for all those living with the effects of brain injury,

and for their families

CONTENTS

PREFACE

ONE OF THE MOST BELOVED and memorable films of all time, the 1939 movie *The Wizard of Oz,* has become an enduring icon of popular culture. Its groundbreaking visuals, comedy, and music mark the film as a masterpiece. An early scene presents a troubling issue that advances the plot. A tornado hits a Kansas farmhouse and a window sash strikes the young heroine, Dorothy, who falls onto her bed, briefly unconscious. When her eyes open, the house is spinning, and then it makes a crash landing in the Land of Oz, where Dorothy and her dog, Toto, begin their adventures. As a child watching this movie, I thought Dorothy was dreaming, but as an adult I understand the fictional Dorothy has sustained a concussion.

In the 1930s and the decades following, films and other media have depicted concussions such as Dorothy's as transient, just a brief jolt to the head. Slapstick comedians bonk heads, and falling anvils flatten cartoon characters, who bounce back instantly. Video games depict either inconsequential or lethal events from head trauma, without much in between. Victims who don't die "see stars," but they quickly recover. These portrayals convey the message—stored in our consciousness as children and young adults—that a concussion is a trivial matter with no lasting consequences.

As a physician, I have heard many concussion stories, but I have been especially struck by the number of serendipitous conversations I have had about concussion during the writing of this book with people who were not my patients. A college friend told me that she fell off a rocking horse at the age of 3. After the incident she remained "in a coma" for a day but fully recovered. "Do you think the fall may lead to any problems later in life?" she wondered. Another friend recounted that she had a sharp memory prior to having a concussion as a teenager but now needs to write things down to remember them. "Could that have been because of the concussion?" she asked. An acquaintance wondered what I thought about her nephew's newly diagnosed seizure disorder. "Might it be related to his several skateboard accidents?" A woman I encountered while walking my family's French bulldog struck up a conversation with me about her brother-in-law. "Could his dementia be related to the multiple concussions he experienced as a linebacker on his high school football team, like some of the NFL players?"

A focus in the media on sports concussion controversies and the accelerating pace of brain injury research has brought concussion into public view and also likely increased the rate of concussion diagnoses. Yet while this attention has heightened awareness of public health issues and risks for young athletes, the explosion of information has also created more questions than answers.

Sports medicine physician Michael Collins and his colleagues at the University of Pittsburgh conducted a Harris Poll survey in 2015 to determine the extent of people's knowledge about concussion. They found that nine in ten Americans could not define a concussion when given five options. Almost half of those surveyed were un-aware that not all concussions happen during contact sports activities. Only about 30 percent recognized that a concussion does not re-quire a blow to the head, or that concussions can be treated. About one-quarter feared their life would change forever if they had a con-cussion. Only about half of those surveyed had confidence that coaches and school personnel had sufficient concussion education.

I have written this book to provide accessible, accurate, and up-to-date information. I answer typical questions about concussion science and concussion treatment within the limits of current and always-evolving knowledge of the human brain. Whether you have personally suffered a concussion or are a friend or family member of a concussion patient, a medical or care professional, or a coach or caseworker, this book will offer answers.

My Journey

My experience with concussion began in 1985, after my residency in physical medicine and rehabilitation (PM&R) and a fellowship in brain injury medicine. In my inpatient practice, I cared for patients in acute-care hospitals, rehabilitation hospitals, and skilled nursing facilities. These patients had survived the most severe trauma to their brains and bodies. They included people in coma or living with other disorders of consciousness, as well as those who had emerged from coma with severe disabilities. We resuscitated and stabilized patients, treated them in trauma and rehabilitation hospitals, and eventually sent them home, sometimes to return to school or work. Many had visible, permanent effects of trauma and physical and cognitive impairments that clearly limited their function and quality of life.

In contrast, in my outpatient practice, I encountered another group of patients who had experienced one or more concussions.

While these patients had non-life-threatening injuries, they improved slowly, and in some cases they never recovered completely. These less-than-ideal outcomes occurred despite the fact that their injuries fell into the so-called mild category by clinical measures and led them and their families—and their doctors—to expect a full recovery. Their injuries could not be located with X-rays, computerized tomography (CT) scans, or laboratory tests, nor could these injuries be confirmed through a physical examination. Many patients experienced very severe symptoms—pounding headaches, disorienting vertigo (a spinning sensation) and balance problems, debilitating insomnia, tinnitus (ringing or buzzing in the ears), hypersensitivity to light and sound, blurred vision, irritability, and difficulty concentrating, reading, and remembering. Some of these symptoms continued for months or even years, and these patients often had difficulty organizing their days and completing tasks, let alone enjoying life in any way.

In some cases, other medical professionals had dismissed their symptoms as transient, imagined, or feigned and sent them home either without a clear diagnosis or with a diagnosis of mental illness. Yes, anxiety, post-traumatic stress disorder (PTSD), depression, or another mental health condition can cause symptoms similar to those of a concussion. Sometimes having one of these conditions can exacerbate concussion symptoms. But even if patients had another condition, this often did not tell the whole story. Their symptoms seemed to worsen through the actions of those who added insult to injury and failed to acknowledge what patients were experiencing or to offer adequate treatment. Patients with invisible injuries such as concussion often have a mix of physical, cognitive, and emotional symptoms that make diagnosis and treatment challenging. Seeking the underlying cause of symptoms requires enough time for information-gathering, focused treatment, and education about the nature of the injury and its consequences.

A study by Pennsylvania social worker Page Walker Buck and her associates documents patients' descriptions of the care they received after a concussion. They heard many dismissive messages: "Oh, it's four to six weeks. You'll be better. It'll be fine. It's all good. Just go home, rest, do not push yourself . . . . Your CAT scans are normal. You know, give it a month. It'll be fine." These messages are similar to those recounted by my patients over decades in clinical practice. The fact that this unhelpful messaging continues is cause for concern. The authors noted: "Research participants were acutely aware that mTBI [mild traumatic brain injury] patients who had been referred for rehabilitation services need more than just rest or a motivational shove. Too often, they found that their patients were left to manage without proactive medical care to provide accurate information about the complexity or anticipated duration of symptoms related to mTBI."

I frequently hear the question, "When will my symptoms go away?" The truth is that we medical professionals are not great at predicting recovery from concussion. We should not presume that we can reliably forecast what will happen to people. Nor should we minimize the symptoms people experience or fail to provide pertinent information about their injuries. Because we still do not have a laboratory biomarker or other determinant that always and definitely proves a concussion has occurred or predicts what recovery will look like, the best approach is careful history-gathering and physical examination, backed by an understanding of the brain, the muscles and nerves, and the physical and psychological consequences of trauma. And despite our inability to clearly pinpoint a diagnosis, we can offer symptomatic treatments, rehabilitation interventions, and self-management strategies that can be very effective in the short and long term.

A recent study, Transforming Research and Clinical Knowledge in Traumatic Brain Injury (TRACK-TBI), led by researcher Seth Seabury at the University of California, San Francisco, found that most people with concussions who are evaluated and treated in emergency rooms (ERs) received no follow-up care. Everyone with a history of concussion should be evaluated, and patients should receive follow-up care if their symptoms do not resolve quickly. Unfortunately, even those who receive adequate acute care may not receive a complete diagnosis, education, or effective and ongoing treatment.

One concussion appears to increase the risk of another. Multiple concussions, whether from sports- and recreation-related activities, a work injury, military service, domestic violence, or other causes, set up a progression of brain events that can lead to devastating consequences in some individuals. Robert Stern, a neurologist at Boston University's Chronic Traumatic Encephalopathy (CTE) Center, testified to the United States Congress in 2017 about the association between neurodegenerative diseases and repetitive concussions. He said, "I do fear we are going to see a very shocking number of people over the next few decades."

The Numbers

The Greek physician Hippocrates, born about five centuries before the Common Era (BCE), describes concussion in the medical and surgical text *De Vulneribus Capitis* (Wounds in the Head) as a state that occurs after a head injury with losses of speech and hearing. The term *commotio cerebri* (shaken brain), a synonym for concussion that has been used for centuries in medical texts, still appears in the World Health Organization's *International Classification of Diseases.*

According to WHO, about half of the global population will experience one or more concussions during their lifetime.

Current annual estimates are that about 70 million people somewhere in the world will experience a traumatic brain injury (TBI), and most of these are concussions or milder brain injuries. This is likely an underestimation because of inadequate reporting methods in many countries, including the United States. Christopher Gaw and Mark Zonfrillo of Brown University reported that 10.7 million people were treated for head trauma in US emergency rooms from 2007 to 2011, a higher number than in previous studies. Concussions increased by almost 38 percent over those five years, and almost a third were sports-related. The largest rate increases were in children younger than 11 years and adults older than 65 years of age.

The US Centers for Disease Control and Prevention (CDC) reports that fall-related TBIs now cause more than 40 percent of all TBIs in the United States, replacing motor vehicle crashes as the leading cause. Falls cause the majority of TBIs in the United States for children from infancy to age 4 and for adults 65 and older. Close to a quarter of all TBIs in children younger than 15 are related to blunt trauma (striking or being struck by an object that is not sharp or penetrating). In many other parts of the world, motor vehicle crashes are still the major cause of TBIs.

In the United States, about 44 million youth participate in sports annually, and about half of all sports- and recreation-related concussions occur in children and adolescents. Boys and girls playing collision and high-contact sports experience the highest incidence of sports concussions and repeat or recurrent concussions. In a CDC study led by Kelly Sarmiento and her colleagues, football, bicycling, basketball, playground activities, and soccer topped the list of activities with the highest ER rates. In high school sports, concussion rates are highest for football and girls' soccer.

A recent study of students in grades 8, 10, and 12 by University of Michigan researchers Phil Veliz and colleagues found that almost 20 percent reported having had a concussion at some point in their lives. Lara DePadilla and colleagues reported in the CDC's *Morbidity and Mortality Weekly Report* in June 2018 that on the Youth Risk Behavior Survey of US high school students, 15 percent of students reported having had a concussion in the twelve months prior to the survey, and 6 percent reported two or more concussions. Male students and students playing team sports reported more concussions than females or those playing non-team sports. The odds of having a concussion increased as the number of sports played increased. Black and Hispanic students were more likely to report four or more concussions than were white students. Twelfth graders were less likely to report a concussion than those in lower grades.

Over the last twenty years, about 2.5 million service men and women have been deployed to Iraq and Afghanistan, and the US military refers to blast injuries as the signature wound of these wars. Operation Enduring Freedom (OEF) began in Afghanistan in October 2001, Operation Iraqi Freedom (OIF) in May 2003, and Operation New Dawn (OND) in Iraq in August 2010. According to the US Department of Defense, more than 375,000 service members have been diagnosed with a TBI since 2000, and more than 100,000 have entered the Veterans Health Administration system of care. About 75 percent of these wartime injuries result from improvised explosive devices (IEDs), land mines, dynamite, bombs, mortars, and grenades.

There are other vulnerable populations that we must not overlook. Eve Valera, a clinical psychologist and researcher at Harvard, has been studying victims of domestic violence (now termed intimate partner violence). She estimated in an MRI study commentary that 1.6 million women suffer repeated TBIs from this violence every year. We have no reliable numbers to report on TBIs in home-less and prison populations, or even reliable TBI records for work-place injuries, for that matter.

Recovery?

For decades, conventional wisdom has held that as few as 5 to 10 percent of people who experience a concussion have symptoms that turn into a chronic condition called post-concussion syndrome (PCS). However, that percentage appears to be increasing.

A 2016 NPR-Truven study found that one-quarter of Ameri-cans reported having a concussion at some point in their lives, and close to 30 percent said they have suffered from long-term effects, most commonly headaches. More than half of this group reported having had more than one concussion. About one in five people in the study did not seek medical care when they had the concussion. In a US TRACK-TBI study, Paul McMahon and colleagues found that eight out of ten patients who had experienced a concussion re-ported at least one post-concussion symptom at six months and again twelve months later. Matthew Eisenberg and his colleagues at Boston Children's Hospital found that patients between the ages of 11 and 22, and those with a previous concussion (and especially those with a history of multiple concussions), were at risk for pro-longed symptoms.

Canadian researchers Charles Tator, Carmen Hiploylee, and their colleagues also found that more than one concussion was as-sociated with a poorer outcome. In the PCS group they studied (ages 10 to 74), 75 percent reported a history of more than one con-cussion. On average, post-concussion symptoms in the group lasted seven months, but 12 percent of people had symptoms lasting more than two years. The number of initial symptoms predicted the dura-tion of PCS, and the average number of chronic symptoms was eight. The most common were headaches, memory deficits, concentration difficulties, imbalance, and dizziness. Approximately one-quarter of the group with PCS had a previous psychiatric condition, attention deficit disorder / attention deficit hyperactivity disorder (ADD / ADHD), a learning disability, or previous migraine headaches. The Canadian research group found in a subsequent study that only 27 percent of the PCS group eventually recovered, and two-thirds of those who recovered did so within the first year. No patients who had PCS lasting three years or longer recovered.

New Zealand researcher Alice Theadom and her colleagues analyzed a database of people older than 16 that included assessments of mood, cognition, and symptoms following a concussion. They found that almost half experienced symptoms related to the concussion one year later. Their levels of anxiety and depression or a reduced quality of life were comparable to the general population, but 11 percent had significant cognitive problems. A history of living alone, using alcohol, having one or more other medical problems, and being female or from a nonwhite ethnic group were predictors of a worse outcome at one year. This research group found that cognitive symptoms and lack of community participation continued for many of those who did not recover.

There is, however, some good news for very young children who experience concussions. In a study by Vicki Anderson and colleagues in Australia, those in a group aged two to seven did well at ten years. Not surprisingly, preinjury abilities and family functioning were predictors of better outcomes for this study's subjects.

This book details what happens in the human brain when it is injured. Neuroscience is still in its infancy, and medicine is an imperfect science. Humans and their brains differ, and they react differently to trauma depending on the nature and circumstances of the injury, pre-injury medical and psychological factors, genetics, age, birth sex or gender, and other factors. The patient stories I recount represent the wide range of scenarios in which head injuries and concussions occur, serving as a set of touchstones for discussing concussion and its diagnosis, treatment, and prevention. I have changed names and other identifying details in order to protect patient privacy.

Part One describes the science of concussion, diagnosis and treatment of concussion and PCS, and the potentially dire consequences of repeat concussions. We know that the human brain responds poorly when it receives too many insults, especially over relatively short periods of time, even if the injury is labeled "minor" or "minimal" or "mild." Medicine can provide symptom relief (often), disease management (sometimes), and cures (rarely). Concussion medicine can currently offer symptom relief but not disease management, and certainly not a cure.

Part Two addresses sports and recreation activities and their associated risks for concussion. Despite substantial evidence of the deleterious effects of repeat hits to the brain, we continue to elevate sports prowess and to subject young people to repeated concussions in popular sports and recreational activities. We are not good at predicting who will have a bad outcome, but that is exactly why we should have better concussion prevention strategies, especially for young people whose brains are still developing. There are many ways to participate in activities that can improve our health and well-being without high concussion risks.

Part Three offers information about other vulnerable populations—the young and the elderly, workers in certain occupations, victims of intimate partner violence and child abuse, prisoners and the homeless, and military personnel. These unique populations have unique needs. Much of our attention has been focused on people with sports- and recreation-related concussions, but these are not the only groups whose needs we must address. We require considerably more scientific and clinical research funding and clinical care for all these populations.

Part One

An Imperfect Science

We look for medicine to be an orderly field of knowledge and procedure. But it is not. It is an imperfect science, an enterprise of constantly changing knowledge, uncertain information, fallible individuals, and at the same time lives on the line. There is science in what we do, yes, but also habit, intuition, and sometimes plain old guessing. The gap between what we know and what we aim for persists. And this gap complicates everything we do.

—ATUL GAWANDE, 2002

1

What Happens to the Brain?

Jason, an emergency room (er) physician I treated in my outpatient clinic, experienced a concussion when he fell from his mountain bike at the age of 42. When he regained consciousness, he realized he must have hit the ground hours before, because his cell phone told him it was early evening. He remembered eating lunch but recalled nothing about his day beyond that. Despite a gash on his forehead and trouble focusing his eyes, he managed to drive himself home. Jason was on ER duty the next day, and he asked his colleagues to order imaging studies. He was certain there was nothing serious to discover, even though he had a pounding headache and felt dizzy when he moved quickly. Jason had always thought the brain got shaken up but not really injured during a concussion. He was sure he would have a full recovery within a few days, even though his symptoms were intense.

For several months, Jason continued to experience intense headaches, dizziness, and insomnia. He had difficulty focusing on his
work, and he felt a combination of physical and mental fatigue. He
wondered what was going on in his brain at the invisible, microscopic level to produce these persistent symptoms. What forces
caused the concussion, and how were those neurons and other cells
reacting? He wondered why he felt worse over the initial weeks and
months, and then very, very slowly better, until his symptoms resolved. Jason had studied the brain in medical school courses, and he
had extensive training in trauma to the brain and body, but now he
had a very personal reason to go back to the books again.

Biology, Chemistry, and Physics

Every patient I have ever cared for has these same questions about
the connections between their lingering symptoms after a concussion. An article entitled "Neurophysiology of Concussion" by Nigel
Shaw, a physiologist from New Zealand, opens with this statement:
"Cerebral concussion is both the most common and most puzzling
type of traumatic brain injury." From there, Shaw lays out his theory
about the science of concussion. He believes that a concussion is a
petit mal type of seizure that involves a loss of memory. Shaw's
theory didn't get much traction when it appeared. However, his
contribution explains two major problems confronting concussion
researchers. He posited first that the "biomechanical events set up by
the concussive blow may ultimately result in stretching, tearing,
compression, or deformation injuries to the neural tissue." Then
he goes on: "Disentangling which one, or combination of these
factors is ultimately responsible for initiating a state of concussion
has proven an arduous task."

Shaw identifies the second problem facing researchers as "the
relationship between transient concussion and more severe kinds of

brain injury in which the period of coma is prolonged." And he asks whether concussion's effects on the brain are unique or whether they "just differ quantitatively from the more severe types of head trauma?" While neuroscience has not fully answered that question, Jason nevertheless wanted to read more about the science of concussion and the controversies surrounding it. What caused him to lose consciousness? Why did he lose awareness and memory? Why did his head feel as though his brain was hurting? Would the injury be permanent?

In what follows, we'll describe what may have happened to Jason's brain during and after his injury that may have produced the symptoms he experienced. The science of concussion draws from neuroscience—cytology (cell biology), biomechanics (the study of structure, function, and movement related to biological systems), biochemistry (the study of chemical processes within biological systems), and neuroanatomy (anatomy of the nervous system)—and began more than a century ago. Neuroscience researchers have often used animal models, making it difficult to draw conclusions about humans. For patients like Jason, we can only speculate about the details. Neuroscience is still in its infancy as a science, and therefore so is concussion science.

Cell Biology

In 1906, Spanish pathologist Santiago Ramón y Cajal and Italian pathologist Camillo Golgi jointly won the Nobel Prize in Physiology or Medicine for their work on the structure of the nervous system. Golgi developed staining techniques that Cajal used and improved. Cajal espoused the neuron doctrine, which proposes that neurons operate as discrete autonomous cells conducting electrical signals in only one direction. Cajal reported changes to cells after a brain injury called chromatolysis, and he acknowledged the work of

German researchers who studied *Gehirnerschütterung* (the German word for concussion). He also identified the synapses (the junctions between nerve cells) where transmission of information from one neuron to another occurs.

Much later, in the 1930s and 1940s, neuropathologist Carl Rand and his colleague Cyril Courville published extensive research they conducted at the Cajal Laboratory of Neuropathology in Southern California, including commentary on the cellular effects of concussion. They reopened long-standing debates with this statement: "The cell changes, it became clear, can be found long after a patient has recovered consciousness, so these changes cannot be responsible for the acute manifestations of concussion. While there is no known way to evaluate the physiologic counterpart of these structural changes clinically, it is possible that they may account for some of the psychic alterations that so often occur after commotio cerebri [shaken brain]."

Rand and Courville concluded that these cellular changes "furnish reason for caution in describing all such manifestations as being purely functional in character." They concluded that earlier researchers failed to see the lasting effects: "It is obvious that these investigators have only segregated the minor alterations in transitory states from more enduring ones and have further contributed to the highly artificial conception of concussion as a purely momentary clinical state." In other words, these renowned basic scientists viewed the cell changes as structural. At the same time, they believed that these changes may be accompanied by functional (not altering to structures, and not permanent) abnormalities that laboratory methods available to them might not reveal. The term "functional," implying a brief disruption of cellular or bodily systems, will continue to crop up in current debates about concussion and concussion guidelines. This use of "functional" and "structural" confused Jason, a physician with extensive medical education and training who was frequently critical of medicine's lack of precision.

Biomechanics

When Jason catapulted from his bicycle on a mountain slope, his body accelerated as his speed increased, and then abruptly decelerated when he landed, hitting the rock. Forces moved his brain around inside his skull. When his brain was shaken, the force injured the neurons, and especially their axons (long processes of nerve cells that conduct impulses to the end of the neuron), affecting the network that carries information from one neuron to another. These forces can disrupt and destroy the stability of myelin, the insulating membrane that surrounds axons.

Beginning in the 1930s, British researcher Sabina Strich pushed brain injury investigations. She studied stretch injuries to axons during acceleration / deceleration events similar to Jason's crash. Strich called her microscopic findings "retraction balls" (swelling of axons), and she surmised that disruption to the flow of cytoplasm (jelly-like fluid inside the cell) caused them. She saw these effects after concussions and after more severe brain injuries. Strich credited physicist A. H. S. Holbourn with describing the impacts of rotational forces on brain tissues during trauma. Holbourn designed simple experiments using physical models with gelatin molds in the 1940s. Disruption of the flow of cytoplasm within the cell body and axon and the formation of retraction balls were important cellular findings in what came to be called diffuse axonal injury (DAI).

In 1945, Northwestern University researchers William Windle and Richard Groat published results of their team's concussion experiments, showing alteration in the shape, size, and arrangements of what are called Nissl bodies. Nissl bodies represent the endoplasmic reticulum (a maze within the cell that moves proteins and other substances), with its ribosomes (the nerve cell's protein factories). The Nissl bodies in their experiments were chromophilic (they "love a stain" and pick up a color). They became visible almost immediately after what these researchers called "rather light blows to the head."

Windle and Groat observed that starting the second day after injury and progressing to a maximum degree at six to eight days, neurons, and in particular, interneurons (connecting neurons) died. They also conjectured about subconcussive injuries (concussion of the brain without obvious signs): "It seems likely that an occasional neuron may disappear even after a subconcussive blow." They went on to say: "it is inconceivable that extreme degenerative changes involving ballooning of the cell and complete loss of Nissl substance can be reversible. Nevertheless, no direct proof has been offered that such altered nerve cells die and disappear after concussion. We cannot fully understand postconcussional behavioral changes until we know whether structural damage is permanent." The endoplasmic reticulum and its ribosomes, which early researchers labeled with Nissl stains, may hold a clue to the mechanism by which repetitive brain injuries lead to neurodegenerative diseases such as chronic traumatic encephalopathy (CTE) (see Chapter 4).

After an axon is injured, further degeneration can occur over time as the axon dies back from its most distant point toward the neuron cell body, a process called Wallerian degeneration. The dendrites (string-like projections at the end of the axon that provide the chemical connections at the synapses) are also vulnerable to violent shaking. The forces that create disruption to these cellular systems cascade over hours, weeks, and even months. It is possible that these microscopic events following the initial concussion caused the symptoms that Jason was experiencing—headaches, sensitivity to light and sound, dizziness, and problems with balance, concentration, and memory.

Figure 1 shows three neurons. The neuron on the left is intact and contains a cell body, an axon, and dendrites. The neuron in the middle shows more detail: the axon's myelin sheath (insulation), microtubules (structural supports) inside the axon, and a cell body. On the far left are two boxes. In the upper box is an enlarged view of the cell body with some of its organelles—the nucleus (containing genetic material), mitochondria (energy centers for the cell), and Nissl substance (the endoplasmic reticulum). In the lower box is a synapse (the gap between neurons) and neurotransmitters (chemical messengers). The neuron on the right depicts a retraction ball and microglial cells (helper cells) activated at the scene of the injury.

Beginning in the 1970s, key US and European laboratories ramped up research on traumatic brain injury (TBI). Hume Adams and David Graham at the University of Glasgow, and Ayub Ommaya and Thomas Gennarelli at the University of Pennsylvania, collaborated with their research teams to show that rotational forces, and resistance to changes in speed or direction of movement, are the primary causes of shear injuries, stretching, and compression strains within the brain. Shear injuries occur through the application of opposing forces, in a direction parallel to a surface, during rapid acceleration and deceleration. Over subsequent decades, University of Pennsylvania and Glasgow colleagues continued this DAI research.

A Brain Injury Grading System

Centuries ago, the brain's white and gray matter could be seen with the naked eye in postmortem brains. In the living brain, blood cells actually render gray matter a pinkish color. Gray matter contains numerous cell bodies, glial cells, dendrites, and axon terminals and synapses, but few myelinated (insulated) axons. In contrast, white

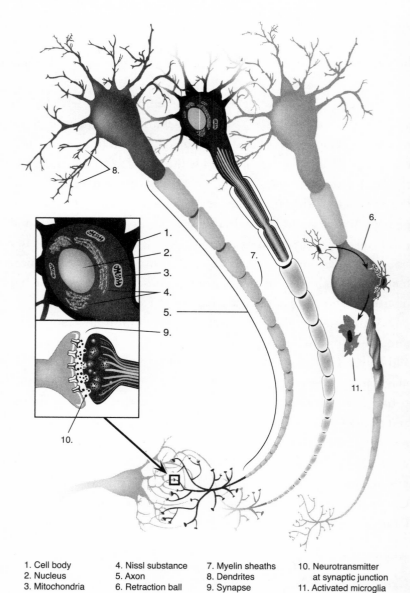

1. Cell body
2. Nucleus
3. Mitochondria
4. Nissl substance
5. Axon
6. Retraction ball
7. Myelin sheaths
8. Dendrites
9. Synapse
10. Neurotransmitter at synaptic junction
11. Activated microglia

FIGURE 1 Two intact neurons and an injured neuron (*right*) with a retraction ball and activated microglial cells. Labels identify internal structures. Insets represent an enlarged view of the cell body, with some of its organelles (*above*) and the synaptic junction (*below*).

matter consists of myelinated axons and axon tracts connecting different parts of gray matter to each other, and white matter contains fewer cell bodies. The different densities of gray and white matter contribute to shear injuries. The corpus callosum, the huge system of white matter tracts connecting the two hemispheres of the brain, is very susceptible to stretching by external forces. The term DAI implies that there is injury everywhere throughout the brain, but that is not what happens. Some researchers and clinicians prefer the term traumatic axonal injury (TAI).

In the 1980s, the Glasgow research team found on autopsies that the pattern of axonal injury and the associated injury to tiny blood vessels correlates with the severity of TBI. Figure 2 depicts this DAI grading system. A Grade I DAI involves the frontal and temporal lobes, and less commonly the parietal and occipital lobes, deep motor systems, or the cerebellum. Jason's magnetic resonance imaging (MRI) scan showed evidence of a Grade I DAI. There were hypodensities (areas of lower density representing damage) in a few areas of the frontal lobes that likely explained his problems with concentration, memory, and information processing.

A Grade II injury additionally involves the corpus callosum, the white matter tracts connecting the two sides of the brain. People with Grade II DAI typically have problems like Jason's, just more severe. A Grade III injury involves the brainstem in addition to the Grade I and II anatomic areas. Many patients with a Grade III injury will be in coma or a prolonged state of unconsciousness.

The DAI system is still utilized in clinical practice because MRI scans can identify the same pattern in the various areas of the brain, providing a measure of severity after TBI. Esther Yuh and her TRACK-TBI (Transforming Research and Clinical Knowledge in Traumatic Brain Injury) study investigators showed the prognostic value of early MRI scans in a group of patients with mild TBIs.

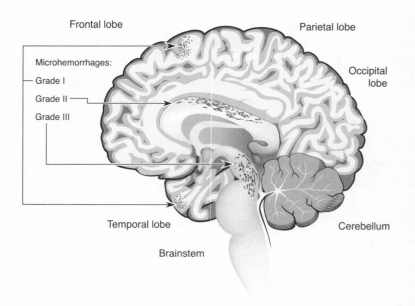

FIGURE 2 The diffuse axonal injury (DAI) grading system developed by Glasgow researchers in the 1980s, based on patterns of microhemorrhages in the brain.

However, because most patients with concussions do not undergo MRI studies, the small microbleeds and other DAI findings that may have occurred after a concussion remain undiscovered. Later, there may be hemosiderin deposits (iron from blood products) on MRI scans, a tell-tale sign of DAI.

Biochemistry

The disrupted biochemistry of TBI involves many chemicals, in both intracellular (inside the cell) and extracellular (outside the cell) spaces. Various toxic and inflammatory substances triggered by a brain injury continue to be suspects and targets of investigation. For example, myelin debris from DAI may activate inflammation and prevent repair of neurons. Alan Faden and David Loane and their colleagues at the University of Maryland and John Povlishock and his team at the Virginia Commonwealth University have studied this toxic cellular environment for many decades. The chemical soup contains calcium and calpain (a protease that breaks down protein) and other contributors to cellular death and apoptosis (programmed cell death).

David Hovda has led other major research efforts at the University of California, first in San Francisco (UCSF) and then in Los Angeles (UCLA). Along with John Povlishock and his colleagues, Hovda's lab is credited with finding evidence of a "window of vulnerability" after concussion. Hovda and his colleagues have been investigating the relationship between concussion symptoms such as migraine headaches and what happens in the brain at the molecular level. A cellular phenomenon called spreading depression (a wave of cellular depolarization, or change in electrical charge, in the brain) may provide the link.

Researchers have also examined the role of the neurotransmitter surge in the brain and cerebrospinal fluid after trauma. For example, Hovda's lab and Yoichi Katayama's research team at UCSF documented the toxicity of glutamate (a widespread, excitatory neurotransmitter). Ronald Hayes and his colleagues at the University of Texas investigated acetylcholine, a neurotransmitter that affects muscles and nerves and plays a role in memory. A reduction in neurotransmitters can result in cognitive disorders and mood disorders such as depression, problems we often see after injuries to the brain. Even Jason's upbeat personality was replaced by some depressive symptoms.

The blood–brain barrier regulates brain chemistry. It is composed of a network of cells, with openings for molecules to pass through. This network controls the movement of beneficial substances such as oxygen and nutrients. Substances such as bacteria and toxins can move through the barrier at times, for example, when it has been damaged during a concussion. Even with milder brain injuries, decreases in blood flow and blood clots can affect the blood-brain barrier.

The brain's supportive cells—the glial cells (astrocytes, oligo-dendrocytes, and microglial cells)—play a role in the concussion story. Damage occurs to these cells and to the vascular endothelium (blood vessel lining) cells that form part of the blood-brain barrier. Astrocytes attach to blood vessels and become activated when an injury occurs. These cells are abundant throughout the central nervous system and migrate to the area of injury, becoming scavenger (clean-up) cells. However, astrocytes also participate in the production of scars that can impede the growth of neurons. Oleksii Shandra and co-investigators at Virginia Tech University found evidence in laboratory rats that scarring produced by astrocytes may set the stage for seizure disorders after repetitive concussions. With a history of only one concussion, however, Jason's risk of developing a seizure disorder was low.

Astrocytes are also active in repair processes such as buffering glutamate, the sometimes-toxic neurotransmitter, regulating blood-brain barrier permeability, and remodeling synapses. Microglial cells release chemicals that promote inflammation, such as cytokines, tumor necrosis factor alpha, and other toxic substances. But like astrocytes, they probably have both beneficial and detrimental effects on neurons after a TBI. Microglial cells use phagocytosis (chewing up of cells) to clean up debris after an injury. Oligodendrocytes, another type of glial cell, are required for repair—the remodeling and remyelination—of the axon.

The glymphatic system is a waste clearance system in the brain that uses a network of channels around blood vessels, believed to be formed by astroglial cells, to transport waste. The glymphatic system may also help distribute other substances in the brain such as glucose, lipids, amino acids, and neurotransmitters. This system functions mainly during sleep and is for the most part inactive while we are awake. The biological need for sleep across all species may reflect the need for the brain to eliminate potentially toxic waste products, including amyloid beta protein (Aβ), which is implicated in Alzheimer's disease. This system therefore has relevance to sleep (Chapter 3) and to neurodegenerative diseases (Chapter 4).

Teasing out the beneficial and detrimental aspects of various cellular and chemical activities challenges researchers trying to find treatments. Jason noted that he had good days and bad days, though not necessarily for any reason he could identify. Altogether, he felt he was getting better over the weeks and months after his injury. It made sense to him that there was inflammation in his brain and then some cleanup; this explanation provided a reason for optimism.

Forces to Reckon With

Biomechanical forces are at play in every TBI, and researchers are discovering more about these forces and concussions. Jason's helmet sported several dents, making it likely that different forces set the stage for his concussion. Two types of external forces can produce a concussion: static loading, when the head is stationary as force is applied; and dynamic loading, when the body or the head is in motion during an impact. Blunt force simply means that an unsharp object strikes the head or the head strikes such an object. Shaking of the brain from whatever cause produces acceleration and deceleration forces leading to internal impacts, without blunt force. Jason's brain experienced what is termed dynamic loading, because he was in motion during the impact. His helmet protected him from a skull fracture and a more severe brain injury, but he still had a risk of a concussion.

There are two basic directions of motion to consider in concussions. One is called translational or linear movement—moving from Point A to Point B in a straight line. The other is a rotational or angular motion, when the body or the head moves in an arc or circle. Calculating the force of these movements requires measures of speed, velocity, acceleration, and deceleration. Speed is the distance traveled over a certain amount of time, while velocity measures the change of position that occurs over that same time period. Velocity is therefore a vector measurement, meaning that it takes into account the position and direction of movement. Acceleration describes the rate at which an object changes its velocity divided by the distance it travels. If an object is increasing in velocity, it's accelerating, and if it's decreasing in velocity, it's decelerating. To repeat a critical point: acceleration–deceleration forces can damage the brain even without a head impact occurring.

We measure linear head acceleration in meters per second, but researchers use g-forces (gravitational forces) for measurement. One g equals 9.8 meters (or 32 feet) per second. These g-forces have been studied on the athletic field and in other settings, and researchers have uncovered some comparative data. We are all subjected to small g-forces daily, but concussions typically occur when the g-force reaches about 100. Figure 3 shows the comparative values for common situations where g-forces are at work.

Isaac Newton's laws of motion come to mind as we picture Jason hurtling down the trail on his bike. First, an object tends to keep moving in a straight line at constant speed: force = mass (m) × acceleration (a). The mass of Jason's head, body, and bicycle join with his rate of acceleration to produce the g-force (g) of his head hitting the ground. Jason's head may have first slammed into the large rock

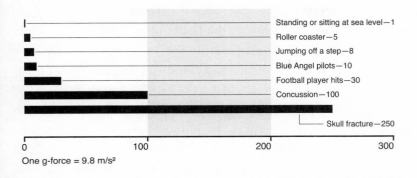

Standing or sitting at sea level—1
Roller coaster—5
Jumping off a step—8
Blue Angel pilots—10
Football player hits—30
Concussion—100

Skull fracture—250

0   100   200   300
One g-force = 9.8 m/s²

FIGURE 3 A comparison of various g-forces that are at play during various human activities.

and then onto the ground. At 5 feet 8 inches tall and weighing approximately 170 pounds, Jason may have incurred around 100–200 g to his brain over 3 milliseconds when his 10-pound head hit the rock at 15 miles an hour, so about 2,000 pounds of force pummeled his brain. If the g-force had been stronger and if he hadn't been wearing a helmet, Jason might have had a skull fracture and a more severe brain injury, not gotten home that night, and possibly not survived.

Rotational acceleration is measured in radians (a circular measurement) per second squared (rad/s²). Research by Steven Rowson and his colleagues at Virginia Tech suggests that these accelerations, ranging from 4,500 to 5,500 rad/s², can inflict a concussion. In combat, collision sports, and other activities where human bodies risk concussions like Jason's, complex rotational forces are obviously at work.

Bird Brains

For decades, scientists and engineers have wondered why woodpeckers don't have brain injuries. As a woodpecker's beak drills into wood, it creates a force in the range of 1,000 g, ten times higher than the 80–100 g that fells football players. These relentlessly pecking birds take thousands of hits to the head every day. For this reason, the woodpecker's head and brain design have been the subject of research for helmet and other technologies for decades.

Birder and commentator Mike O'Connor wrote a book called *Why Don't Woodpeckers Get Headaches?*, a question that a sixth grader asked him. An answer lies in the highly developed horseshoe-shaped hyoid bone which protects the bird's brain. O'Connor found that the woodpecker's "extra-long tongue wraps around inside the back of the woodpecker's head. When the bird wants to reach deep into a tree for a tasty insect treat, it shoots out its tongue like one of those annoying party favors." This long sliver of soft bone—the hyoid bone—functions both as an unusual tongue and as a seat belt for the bird's brain. Humans also have a hyoid bone that anchors our tongue and plays a role in swallowing and speech. But our hyoid bone—a bone most people have never heard of—does not serve as a tethering strap for our brains as it does for woodpecker brains. If it did, we might not be as vulnerable to concussion.

In the 1970s, Phillip May and his UCLA colleagues speculated that a woodpecker's drilling involves linear rather than rotational forces, making it less damaging to bird brains. However, Boston University ornithologist George Farah and his colleagues recently discovered microscopic evidence of the neurodegenerative disease CTE in some pecking birds. Were those particular bird brains subjected to rotational forces, or is there another explanation?

Fluid Biomarkers

Biomarkers document injury to cells or components of cells. For example, troponin, a substance found in the blood after cardiac muscle damage, serves as a cardiac biomarker for people with chest pain. Troponin levels in the blood aid in diagnosing a heart attack.

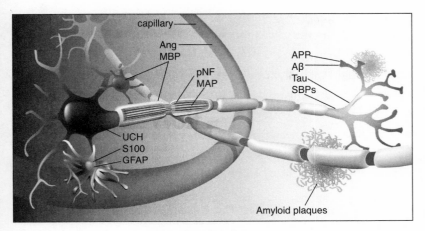

Neuronal cell body:
UCH—ubiquitin carboxyl-terminalhydrolase

Astroglial cell: **S100**—calcium-binding protein;
GFAP—glial fibrillary acidic protein

Myelin sheath and oligodendrocyte:
MBP—myelin basic protein

Capillary: **Ang**—angiopoietin

Axon:
pNF—phosphorylated neurofilament;
MAP—microtubule-associated protein

Axon terminal:
SBPs—spectrin breakdown products;
Tau—tau protein; **APP**—amyloid precursor protein; **Aβ**—amyloid beta;
Amyloid plaques

FIGURE 4 Laboratory biomarkers originating from various parts of the neuron, such as the cell body, axon, myelin, or astrocytes and capillaries.

Scientists are exploring potential fluid biomarkers that would work similarly to connect symptoms and signs to the biology of concussion. Possible sources include blood, saliva, urine, or cerebrospinal fluid, the fluid that bathes the brain and spinal cord. Figure 4 shows a plethora of potential biomarkers from various parts of the neuron, such as the cell body, the axon, and myelin. In 2018, the FDA approved the first two of these biomarkers: glial fibrillary acidic protein (GFAP) and ubiquitin C-terminal hydrolase L1 (UCH-L1), developed by Banyan Biomarkers.

How could such biomarkers help Jason or his ER patients? They might help with diagnosing and measuring the severity of concussions. They may contribute data to inform decisions such as whether a computerized tomography (CT) scan is necessary to rule out a brain hemorrhage. Biomarkers for concussion hold great potential to help with diagnosis and prognosis, especially if they can be combined with neuroimaging studies and clinical data. They may also be used to measure the response to treatment. Further biomarker research is clearly needed. Even after a definitive concussion biomarker or biomarkers are agreed upon by medical scientists, physicians will use additional clinical data for diagnosis or treatment decisions.

Neuroanatomy

Jason's injury showed up on MRI scans in both frontal lobes of his brain. The frontal lobes are the largest, taking up one-third to one-half of the total brain mass. It's odd that they were once called "the silent lobes," because they house important cognitive functions such as thinking and memory in what is called the prefrontal region (the front part of the frontal lobes). They also participate in executive functioning—the capacity to prioritize, organize, and use specific mental abilities that live elsewhere in the brain. The right and left frontal lobes serve as integrative centers for pathways from other parts of the brain. Along with the temporal lobes, the frontal lobes are especially vulnerable to injury from shear forces because of how they are seated on the rough surface at the skull base, the platform the brain sits on inside the head, as well as other anatomical factors.

The primitive limbic system, with its relationship to emotions, learning and memory, motivation, and behavioral control contains various links to the frontal and temporal lobes. The hippocampus, a two-horned structure in the limbic system, lies in the temporal lobes on both sides of the brain and connects with other structures in the limbic system. The hippocampus is known as the brain's librarian, the structure responsible for forming short-term memories, then labeling and storing them for future retrieval (much like a hard drive). Hippocampal stem cells remain undeveloped until they are called into action. Scientists have known for decades that the hippocampus is highly susceptible to any kind of insult or injury, such as physical or psychic trauma or a lack of oxygen. Even when Jason regained consciousness, he was likely in a state of post-traumatic amnesia (PTA) and not remembering—evidence suggesting that the hippocampus was not functioning normally.

Researcher Tara Raam and her colleagues at Harvard University discovered that the hippocampus also plays a role in social memory, the capacity to distinguish a friend from a stranger or enemy, through the neurochemical oxytocin. This research shows promise for understanding autism spectrum disorders, post-traumatic stress disorder (PTSD), and TBI. The amygdalae are a pair of almond-shaped structures in the limbic system at the lower ends of the hippocampus. These neuronal masses are implicated in mood and behaviors provoked by anger, aggression, and fear. (See Chapter 4 for related topics, such as neurodegenerative conditions.)

Sensory processing takes place in many areas of the brain, and the parietal and occipital lobes house higher-level systems for physical sensation, vision, and hearing. The thalamus serves as a relay station for many brain functions and may be more vulnerable to injury in children than adults. Concussion often disrupts visual and vestibular (balance and orienting) systems. We can't neglect the cerebellum, either. This structure was once considered only a part of the motor and balance system of the brain, but we now appreciate its role in complex cognition. The midbrain area of the brainstem houses the reticular activating system (RAS), the anatomic region responsible for our level of alertness. The RAS may be a site of injury when a person loses consciousness, for example when Jason blacked out as his head hit the rock. The midbrain is also important for eye movements and hearing, and even memory (see Figure 6 below). Using advanced neuroimaging technology, University of Rochester researchers Adnan Hirad and Jeffrey Bazarian and their colleagues found that the midbrains of football players are especially vulnerable to rotational forces during concussion and clinically silent subconcussions.

Over one hundred years ago, German neurologist Korbinian Brodmann first organized the cerebral cortex of the brain into fifty-two sections based on cellular characteristics. While scientists and pathologists still utilize Brodmann's system, we now focus less on the lobes of the brain and more on tracks, or what is called the connectome—the brain circuitry revealed in large part through advanced neuroimaging techniques.

Neuroimaging

CT scans guide a physician's decision-making about hospitalization or early surgical management and provide the best results for evaluating bones, including skull fractures, large hemorrhages, and edema or swelling in the brain and the spine. However, a CT scan might not detect a hemorrhage smaller than five millimeters. If a CT scan reveals evidence of trauma but the clinical information suggests a milder injury or concussion, the physician may use the term "complicated mild brain injury." In other words, the injury and diagnosis are more complicated because of a lack of correlation between the clinical information and the CT scan results. Categorizing mild cases as complicated can be useful for decisions at the acute stage of an injury. However, lesions on CT scans for milder cases may not predict outcomes, as Marianne Lannsjö and her Swedish colleagues found in a large study of patients with mild TBIs followed up at three months after injury.

Because Jason worked in an ER and held a position in the medical hierarchy, he was able to obtain MRI scans the day after his injury which provided evidence that he had suffered a DAI Grade I injury. His hospital wasn't an academic medical center, but it had an MRI scanner that could do a fluid-attenuated inversion recovery (FLAIR) scan. The MRI FLAIR images of Jason's brain revealed abnormalities in spotty areas of his frontal lobes representing tissue damage from DAI. The axons themselves were not visible. Only a microscope could tell that tale.

MRI scans detect injury using measurements of the movement and direction of water molecules. MRI scans can measure what is called lesion load and lesion volume, a quantification of the amount of injury. For example, MRI scans can measure the extent of atrophy (loss of brain matter) of the hippocampus, the memory center. MRI scans can pick up small lesions at higher rates than CT scans, especially shortly following an injury. Most ER physicians do not order MRIs for patients with concussions because they are not thought to help with clinical decision-making. In addition, they are more expensive and not as readily available as CT scans.

The most extensively utilized imaging technology for researching concussions is MRI diffusion tensor imaging (DTI). DTI technology can detect swelling within brain cells in the early period after a concussion, as well as later consequences of injury. Pinpointing injury with DTI to tracks and bundles of axons, the brain's white matter, is called tractography. DTI can detect small lesions within these tracts. DTI research has revolutionized how scientists understand the brain's connectivity, and in particular what happens to white matter tracts after a concussion. DTI is not, however, ready for prime time, because we don't know what all the findings mean and how they relate to symptoms, signs, severity, or recovery. In addition, not all the research findings to date have been consistent.

Figure 5 shows the major white matter tracts in the brain. The huge corpus callosum tract houses more than 200 million nerve fibers that connect the brain's two hemispheres. It communicates information between the hemispheres for various physical and mental functions. Injury can produce problems with coordination and complex mental functions. The anterior corona radiata maintains attentional control so that we do not become distracted, and it is also linked to the brain's limbic system. The cingulate cortex, the hippocampus, and the fornix are parts of the limbic system, and these tracts also play roles in cognition, mood, and behavior. The uncinate fasciculus, the tract that connects the limbic system with the frontal and temporal lobes, also plays a major role in memory retrieval, decision-making, and emotional states.

Psychologist Trevor Wu and his research colleagues in Utah and Texas studied adolescents with normal CT scans but post-concussion symptoms after a mild brain injury using DTI. They found that damage to the cingulate cortex correlated with memory problems. Lea Alhilali and her colleagues at the University of Pittsburgh found through DTI studies a link to post-concussion symptoms of two types—visual (focusing of the eyes on a near point) and vestibular (balance and equilibrium).

Jason had difficulty with concentration and working memory—the ability to hold on to and manipulate new information in his head—cognitive tasks that were critical to his work as an ER physician. He also had problems organizing and prioritizing his day and organizing his thoughts when he wrote notes into patients' medical records. A DTI MRI scan, had the technology been available for Jason, might have shown detailed white matter tract abnormalities in his brain related to his cognitive difficulties and physical symptoms.

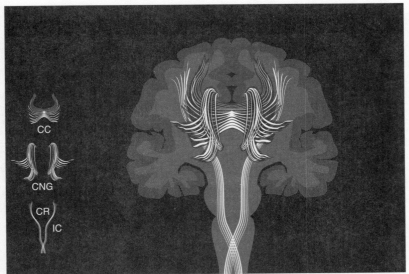

anterior coronal view

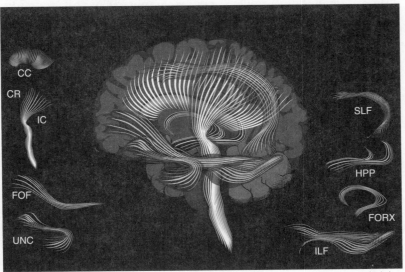

sagittal view

CC—*Corpus callosum;* **CR**—*Corona radiata;* **CNG**—*Cingulate cortex;* **UNC**—*Uncinate fasciculus;* **HPP**—*Hippocampus;* **IC**—*Internal capsule;* **SLF**—*Superior longitudinal fasciculus;* **FORX**—*Fornix;* **FOF**—*Fronto-occipital fasciculus;* **ILF**—*Inferior longitudinal fasciculus*

FIGURE 5 Major white matter (axonal) tracks and their connections throughout the brain.

Some research institutions make available advanced neuroimaging studies to their physicians, but when studies are performed under research guidelines, patients may not be identified, except by a number. High cost and a lack of substantial clinical correlations have prevented these studies from being available to patients, but over time, guidelines change, and availability and access to care and imaging technologies improve. With this progress, patients will receive more diagnostic and predictive data from their physicians.

Athlete Brains

Using neuroimaging to study concussion has opened the door to preliminary evaluations of what happens in the neurons of concussed athletes. For example, Stephano Signoretti and his laboratory colleagues in Rome used MRI technology to investigate disruptions of energy production and metabolism in cells after concussion. They found that calcium overload in the mitochondria (energy centers of the cell) produces oxidative stress, a process that in turn wreaks havoc on the cell's respiratory system. These MRI techniques help to clarify what happens at the cellular level that may result in the concussion symptoms athletes and others typically experience.

Pennsylvania State University researcher Semyon Slobounov and his collaborators used several MRI techniques to study National Collegiate Athletic Association (NCAA) football players over a season. They demonstrated abnormalities in the cingulate cortex, hippocampus, and other brain regions. Not only did 44 percent of the players show abnormalities, but these players had experienced high g-forces on a daily basis from their sport. Brian Johnson and his Penn State colleagues used MRI spectroscopy (MRS) to study brain chemistry in concussed athletes. They demonstrated reductions in metabolism in those recovering from concussions. Neuroscientist Timothy Meier of the Medical College of Wisconsin and his research team showed that declines in blood flow detected by MRI scanning helped predict poorer recovery after sports concussions.

Jeremy Strain and co-investigators at Washington University and the University of Texas / Southwestern have studied the brains of retired NFL players using MRI technology. Athletes reporting a history of concussion with loss of consciousness, and those with a history of playing more games, were more likely to have cognitive impairments and depression. They were also more likely to have a reduction in the size of the hippocampus on MRI scans. University of Toronto researcher Karen Misquitta and colleagues, in a study that compared control subjects with retired professional athletes, found that the volume of the hippocampus was smaller on MRI scans in those with a history of concussions.

Nathan Churchill and his University of Toronto colleagues conducted advanced imaging studies of athletes who did not report symptoms, but their brain images still showed effects of a recent injury on white matter tracts. Although the researchers screened out any athletes with a prior history of concussion, it is possible the white matter changes resulted from previous injuries or concussions that the athletes did not report. In related studies, Churchill's group showed that athletes who returned to play had persisting changes on imaging studies. Those who took longer to return to play showed brain differences that were related to vision, planning, and movement. Churchill's research group also showed more DTI abnormalities in those athletes playing collision versus other contact sports, and between those playing contact versus noncontact sports.

Disrupted Brain Networks

Floaters (specks, lines, or cobwebs that you see when you move your eyes) are more likely to occur from direct eye trauma or aging than from a concussion, but if this condition occurs after a TBI, it warrants an ophthalmologic evaluation. A complaint of double vision at distance, or unequal pupils, requires an urgent examination to be sure there is not a more serious brain injury involving the cranial nerves (nerves related to functions of the head and eyes) or injury to the orbits (eye sockets) and eye muscles. These cases require imaging of the brain. The usual symptoms after concussion reveal subtle evidence of a brain injury. When the brain is shaken with concussive forces, visual and vestibular systems are often affected. These highly complex and interconnected systems involve reactions and reflexes, eye movements, postural stability, and coordination. When concussion disrupts these systems, symptoms such as dizziness, feeling off-balance, headaches, blurred vision, difficulty focusing when moving the eyes quickly, and even attention and thinking problems can occur. Vestibular physical therapists and neuro-ophthalmologists and neuro-optometrists can contribute to the diagnosis and treatment of these conditions (see Chapter 2). Figure 6 represents some of the potentially disrupted regions and connections that cause these symptoms after a concussion. The figure is both complex and over-simplified, but it highlights the most important systems in concussion science that might explain a patient's symptoms.

Visual stimuli reach the visual cortex in the occipital lobe by traveling along the afferent visual pathway, which includes the optic nerves, optic chiasm, and optic radiations. The visual cortex organizes this information and enables us to appreciate the color, shape, and size of objects. The visual cortex projects this information to other lobes of the brain to give topographic orientation (orientation to the physical environment), object recognition (identification of things by words and memories), and meaning to what we see.

When the eyes track an object either slowly using smooth pursuit eye movements (tracking movements of the eyes), or quick saccadic eye movements (rapid movement of the eyes between fixation

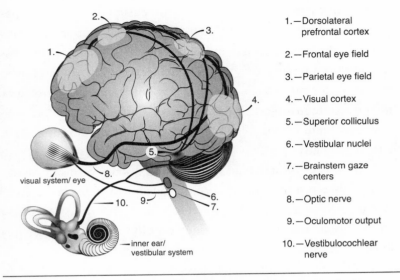

1. — Dorsolateral prefrontal cortex

2. — Frontal eye field

3. — Parietal eye field

4. — Visual cortex

5. — Superior colliculus

6. — Vestibular nuclei

7. — Brainstem gaze centers

8. — Optic nerve

9. — Oculomotor output

10. — Vestibulocochlear nerve

visual system/ eye

inner ear/ vestibular system

FIGURE 6 Key brain regions and pathways that can be disrupted after a concussion. Disruptions can cause problems with vision, hearing, equilibrium, and balance.

points), multiple parts of the brain work to coordinate our eye movements together at the same speed and direction.

Kaiser Permanente neuro-optometrist Jacqueline Theis explained these networks to me: "The visual system is incredibly complex and requires absolute precision. A simple eye movement from side to side requires a different part of the brain than an eye movement up and down. If our eye muscles and the neuronal systems that connect to them are weak, or if injury or disease affects the nerves or neurons involved in coordination of the nerves to the muscles, then double vision may occur. If the complicated network of brain and eye connections is disrupted from a concussion, our eyes may be unable to make smooth pursuits or accurate saccades—eye movements that are essential to tasks like tracking a ball in sports, reading a line of text, or scrolling on a phone."

Jason had trouble reading after his concussion because he experienced problems focusing when reading, and he often felt "off-balance" when moving his head and walking. He had to limit his time on the computer, and he was not able to read his favorite mystery novels for more than about half an hour. Complaints of new difficulty with fluctuating clarity of near vision and discomfort with prolonged reading such as Jason experienced are common after TBI, including concussion.

Jason had both convergence and accommodative insufficiency. Convergence insufficiency is a condition in which the eyes don't work together when looking at a close object, one of the eyes may turn outward, and intermittent double vision may occur. Accommodative insufficiency is a condition in which focusing on objects up close causes near blur. Both conditions are common in 20 to 30 percent of the general population, so these findings are not specific to concussion. However, convergence insufficiency and accommodative insufficiency rates after a TBI are higher than in the general population, suggesting a concussion may cause or worsen these conditions.

A tiny area in the midbrain of the brainstem called the superior colliculus is thought to serve as a sensory integration system that responds to visual, auditory, and other sensory inputs and orients the head toward a stimulus. If you quickly turn your head or jump up and down in Zumba class, your eyes and the balancing centers in your brain adjust just as quickly. The vestibular nuclei make us able to balance and provide our sense of equilibrium. The vestibulocochlear nerve is linked to structures in the ear that sense gravity and position and help to keep us aware of our orientation, remain stable, or stay balanced when we move. Injury to these systems might explain Jason's perception of dizziness when he turned his head quickly, and his sense of being off-balance when he got up quickly from a chair.

The dorsolateral prefrontal cortex (DLPC) is a site for executive functions such as initiating, planning, prioritizing, decision-making, and working memory (remembering and using information at the same time such as while doing a mathematical calculation in your head). Jason's neuropsychology evaluation showed that he had difficulty in these areas of functioning after his injury, resulting in difficulties with the demands of his highly complex job.

Jason also wondered about his mental and physical fatigue. Was it simply due to his problems with insomnia? In 2019, Australian researcher Alan Pearce and his colleagues at La Trobe University found that a technique called transcutaneous magnetic stimulation showed that fatigue and slowed reaction times in patients with post-concussion symptoms were linked to abnormalities in brain networks. Understanding the connection between the disruption of these complex brain networks and their symptoms will help patients like Jason feel reassured that it is not "all in my head."

The Developing Brain

The developing brain differs from the mature brain in water content, myelination and synapses, blood volume, metabolic rates, blood flow, and the shape and elasticity of its skull sutures (junctions between skull bones). Injury to the young brain can impede development, and in some cases arrest or reverse development. Brain maturation occurs in growth clusters at approximately ages 2, 4, 7, 11, 15, and 20 years. We know that the young brain stops expanding in size at about age 5, but reorganization and increased connectivity continue to occur until young people reach their mid- to late twenties. Postural stability and the postural control system typically reach adultlike values between 7 and 10 years of age. These developmental processes occur in a nonlinear fashion.

Ingrid Olsen and her research colleagues at Temple University found through DTI studies that the uncinate fasciculus (see Figure 5) continues to develop into the third decade of life. Although Olsen primarily studies developmental disorders, her research suggests that injury to the uncinate fasciculus may be responsible for some of the cognitive and emotional effects of TBIs. Kristie Whitaker and her colleagues at the University of Cambridge have investigated the map of neural connections—the connectome—in the adolescent brain using MRI scanning techniques. They found evidence of myelination-associated anatomic changes in those aged 14 to 24, evidence of significant human brain growth and remodeling during this decade. The stories of younger brains continue in Chapters 6 and 8.

Not So Simple

We still face many challenges in applying all of this complex scientific and medical information to our understanding of Jason, or of any person with symptoms and signs of a concussion. Much more research is needed to correlate concussion symptoms and signs and disruption of brain networks. In addition, an individual's biological characteristics—birth sex, age, and genetics—may influence how their brain responds to injury and how healing happens. Diagnosing concussion is even more complicated because of the psychological, social, and environmental factors that influence what happens before, during, and after an injury. Chapter 2 focuses on clinical diagnosis for real people, in the context of real-world health care in the twenty-first century.

2

The Search for a Diagnosis

N 1886, the *Boston Medical and Surgical Journal* described the unfortunate case of Louisa Russell. A freight train boxcar struck Russell's house while she cooked in her kitchen in Arlington, Massachusetts. The physician who examined Ms. Russell, Dr. Arthur H. Nichols, testified during the trial that "at the time of crash she was stooping over the oven with her right side toward the wall of the house thus broken in, and avers that she received a blow on the side of her head, after which she was more or less dazed and can give no intelligent account of what occurred, except that she was very much frightened."

The case report, written by Nichols, debates Russell's symptoms, signs, and behavior, then ends with: "In behalf of the defendant it was urged, that the subjective character of the symptoms, the mildness of the local pain, and above all the absence of decided paralysis of the face or extremities, pointed rather to functional disturbance, the sequelae of fright or worry rather than of injury; and that the prognosis was, therefore, favorable. The latter view appears to have found favor with the jury, who awarded the plaintiff the moderate sum of one thousand dollars."

An unfortunately long history shows physicians and other health-care professionals ascribing concussion symptoms to psychiatric causes. Nichols used the term "functional disturbance" in Russell's case to mean that she had a psychological reaction or a transient effect of brain function, rather than a physical or structural injury to her brain. Reading the account now, we can't be sure, but probably Louisa Russell experienced both a concussion and understandable emotional reactions to the sudden crash of a freight train into her house. Who wouldn't have been frightened and worried?

No Intelligent Account

In the 1960s, Oxford University's first neurologist, William Ritchie Russell, concluded from his research that different concussion severities can be measured by the period of post-traumatic amnesia (PTA), trouble remembering things going forward after the injury. Russell described PTA duration as the period of impairment or loss of consciousness, and then any period of amnesia (memory loss) that followed. This gave clinicians a predictive factor not previously available.

William Russell believed that a patient's subjective report of what happened to them proved that an injury to the brain had occurred. He observed that "a distinct qualitative and obvious change in the patient's awareness and orientation is reflected by such questions as, 'Where am I?'; 'What am I doing here?'; or 'What happened?'" Although the events leading up to the injury remain vague to its victim, wrote Russell, "an important qualitative change in mental processes, restoration of the capacity to store current events, can be established by simple tests of recall." Russell also brought to light the concept of retrograde amnesia (the loss of memory for events before the injury), additional evidence that an injury to the brain had occurred. Louisa Russell was unable to give "an intelligent account of what occurred," suggesting that she was in a state of PTA after the train hit her house.

Accident Neurosis

In the 1950s, New York neurologists Peter Denker and Gerald Perry studied patients with a history of concussion, intentionally excluding those like Louisa Russell who were involved in pending or ongoing litigation. In their studies, about 30 percent of patients still had symptoms such as headache, dizziness, and what they called nervous instability at one year after their injury, and about 15 percent continued to have symptoms after three years. Denker and Perry made the case that concussion isn't a trivial event, is likely caused by a brain injury, and that lawyers and examiners "belittled" patients, contributing to their poor outcomes.

A decade after Denker and Perry's work appeared, however, the tables turned on the question of whether post-concussion symptoms were psychiatric rather than neurologic. British neurologist Henry Miller's 1961 article in the *British Medical Journal,* "Accident Neurosis," represented a watershed moment in the debates about what concussion and post-concussion symptoms mean and how they link to litigation and mental health. One of the most influential and widely cited concussion researchers in the 1950s and 1960s, Miller analyzed medico-legal cases in which "gross neurotic symptoms after an accident had been found."

Although Miller did not detail his methodology, as peer-reviewed journals now require, he concluded, "in this series persistence and psychoneurotic elaboration of the post-concussional syndrome bore an inverse relation to the severity of brain injury similar to that observed in the case of frank neurosis." In other words, the less severe the injury, the more likely the person was to develop ongoing post-concussion symptoms that Miller considered neurotic. Among his conclusions, he made this final argument: accident neurosis is cured for most people after they receive a legal settlement.

Medical historian Ryan Ross summarized Miller's research and commentary about the cause of the condition: "Miller postulated that accident neurosis was related to a lack of social responsibility on the part of the claimant, that those claimants with less autonomy in their work, and less of a stake in the fruits of industry, were more likely to develop traumatic sequelae." Ross also concluded that Miller held the medico-legal process responsible for the condition, and he "castigated the medical profession for not properly grasping the problem." Medical historian Stephen Casper conveyed to me that Miller's writing suggests "he had staunchly leftwing views, and that may have made him sympathetic to the plight of workers but unimpressed by their means of resistance."

Other researchers climbed on Miller's bandwagon, suggesting neurosis was responsible, at least in part and in some patients, for post-concussion symptoms. Another British researcher, David Kay, studied a large group of patients in the 1970s and concluded that, although they could not attribute statistical significance, "taken together, psychosocial features discriminated between the groups better than the degree of severity of brain trauma."

In 1977, William Rutherford, an emergency medicine physician in Belfast, Ireland, and his colleagues published the results of a large study of concussed patients that concluded: "While our results could be interpreted as an indication that some patients suffer from organic brain damage and others from post-traumatic neurosis, it seems probable that in many patients there is an interplay of both these elements." In a follow-up study, Rutherford and his colleagues divided patients a year after their injuries into two types, those with symptoms due to neurologic factors that occurred early, and those with symptoms due to psychological factors, which in some cases "prevent the resolution of symptoms" and in other patients "stimulate the production of new symptoms."

Swedish neurologist Hans Lidvall and his colleagues followed patients with mild head injuries over months, and they also concluded that the cause of post-concussion symptoms was complicated, with psychological factors at play.

Do Physicians Cause the Disorder?

In the 1970s and 1980s, British neurologist Reginald Kelly challenged Miller's claims. Kelly studied patients referred to him on average three months after their injury. He showed that symptoms arose in patients who were not pursuing litigation, and that some patients with sports injuries were similarly affected with post-concussion symptoms. He found that settling a claim did not necessarily lead to a resolution of symptoms, as Miller had argued. Kelly and his research colleague, Norman Smith, believed that their studies refuted four myths about post-traumatic syndrome (PTS), the term Miller used for post-concussion symptoms: no one ever recovers and returns to work before a settlement is reached; the condition never occurs if there is no possibility of obtaining compensation or a pension; it never occurs after severe injuries and is always out of proportion to the severity of injury; and it never occurs in "patients of the managerial or professional classes."

Reginald Kelly proposed that PTS was an iatrogenic disease, that is, caused by the actions or behaviors of the medical profession. He believed PTS to be: "perpetuated mainly by the attitude of the medical profession in (1) failing to explain the cause of the symptoms in the first place; (2) either denying their existence or unsympathetically declaring that they are related to the question of compensation; (3) refusing to treat them properly or at all; and (4) declaring that the symptoms will not disappear in any case until the case is settled."

Kelly's research brought him to the conclusion that this attitude of medical practitioners resulted in "many years of lost work, of broken families, due to symptoms which, as I have previously shown and today demonstrated again, frequently respond to prompt, sympathetic and effective treatment." He also argued that actual structural damage to the brain or other anatomic structures causes postconcussion symptoms. He stressed, for example, that vertigo can result from injury to the brainstem, cerebellum, and to the structures of the ear (see Chapter 1, Figure 6).

Kelly emphasized that some patients felt resentment in addition to their list of physical and cognitive symptoms. But he emphasized that "[t]his resentment is compounded when they meet disbelief from the medical profession and the lawyers, a refusal to treat their symptoms, and a vague hint of moral disapproval that they should dare seek compensation for their financial loss." Into the early 1980s he continued to advocate against dismissing the needs of patients. Even contemporary textbooks, he argued, "dismiss this devastating illness." He wrote of PTS as "a condition seen many times by all physicians," in contrast to other conditions that "most physicians never see."

Narrative Medicine

When I did my medical studies and training in the 1970s and 1980s, diagnostic acumen was associated primarily with interviewing the patient, a parent, or a caregiver to learn the symptoms and past medical and surgical conditions and collect other diagnostic data. Called "taking a history," this was taught as a fundamental clinical skill. Once you had completed the history, you conducted a physical examination to confirm the diagnostic hunch you formed during the interview. It was all about thinking it through on the basis of data derived from the patient's story and the examination. The problems patients report (their symptoms) or the abnormalities discovered by an examining physician (called signs) led to a tentative diagnosis. The history elicited is the chronological story of the patient's current chief complaint or primary symptom, and their health- and disease-related experiences. The review of systems is defined as data, especially symptoms, collected from interviewing the patient that relate to bodily functioning.

As with the diagnosis of mental health disorders, the diagnosis of concussion still derives primarily from information gathered by talking with patients. No single symptom or sign by itself supports a diagnosis of concussion. In gathering the history, we must also learn who the patient was before the injury occurred to determine what symptoms may be a consequence of the concussion, which symptoms have worsened, and which may be due to other distinct or related conditions.

Physicians explore additional patient narratives when they conduct the interview in this traditional way. For example, the past medical and surgical history covers what patients have gone through in the way of illnesses, injuries (including previous concussions), and procedures prior to their injury. The family history elicits conditions diagnosed in family members to which the patient may be susceptible. The social history assesses the patient's educational level, employment situation, and social habits, such as whether they use alcohol, tobacco, or other substances, and whether they exercise, any of which might affect their health. Physiatrists and rehabilitation therapists also collect data about the patient's functional abilities to determine what they perceive as activity limitations (for example, reading or stair-climbing) and participation restrictions (for example, difficulty playing golf, taking care of children, or working as an accountant).

Each component of this comprehensive data set leads to a diagnosis of a patient's condition or conditions and provides the basis for determining a comprehensive treatment plan. Because we do not have reliable biomarkers or imaging studies to depend on, this fundamental skill on the part of the physician is still key to the diagnosis of concussion and related symptoms. Unfortunately, in the age of information technology, information about laboratory tests or imaging studies may be available but unhelpful. This old-fashioned history-gathering enterprise is still essential for diagnosis in people with concussions.

Measures of Brain Trauma Severity

In the 1970s, neurosurgeons Bryan Jennett and Graham Teasdale and their colleagues developed the Glasgow Coma Scale (GCS) to assess the severity of a TBI and to identify patients in need of hospitalization or surgery. A GCS score of 13 to 15 indicates a mild TBI, but the Glasgow Scale did not turn out to be as useful for determining severity or outcomes for people with milder injuries as for those with more severe injuries. A perfect GCS score of 15 means the person is awake and alert and communicating, but that score doesn't guarantee a concussion did not occur.

Texas neuropsychologist Harvey Levin and his colleagues developed a brief cognitive scale in the 1970s—the Galveston Orientation and Amnesia Test (GOAT), a measure of PTA, the post-traumatic amnesia that William Russell described in the 1960s. The GOAT can help to predict outcomes and supplements the GCS. A score of equal to or greater than 75 out of 100 on the GOAT for two consecutive days, twenty-four hours apart, means the person is no longer in a state of PTA. There are several versions of the GOAT, including one for children. Unfortunately, very few patients with concussion or even more severe brain injuries are evaluated for PTA using the GOAT, in emergency rooms (ERs) or anywhere else.

The American Congress of Rehabilitation Medicine described mild TBI in the early 1990s with another widely accepted definition: a person has had a mild TBI if they experience a period of loss of consciousness or loss of memory for events immediately before or after an injury, or an alteration in mental state at the time of injury. For an injury to be considered mild, the period of loss of consciousness cannot exceed thirty minutes, and the period of PTA cannot be greater than twenty-four hours, according to this organization's definition. Many patients considered to have mild TBIs based on a GCS of 13 to 15 have periods of PTA much longer than twenty-four hours, as Mark Sherer and his colleagues found. This represents a problem with the American Congress of Rehabilitation's definition.

Loss of consciousness is a poor measure of concussion severity, because most people who have a concussion do not lose consciousness. Patients who do not lose consciousness but have prolonged periods of PTA will often have poorer outcomes than those who lose consciousness but have short periods of PTA. A history of a brief convulsive concussion (a concussion accompanied by a seizure) is also a poor measure of what may happen in terms of recovery. The seizure is a brief and transient event that may not correlate with the extent of trauma to the brain.

To Image or Not to Image the Brain

A former patient of mine, Sarah, fell backward from a playground swing when she was 4 years old. She lost consciousness following a convulsive concussion that lasted for several minutes. An ambulance took Sarah to an ER, and she regained consciousness on the way to the pediatric trauma hospital. At her discharge a couple of days later, she received a clean bill of health. But although she never had another seizure, Sarah always had trouble in school. She was diagnosed with attention deficit disorder / attention deficit hyperactivity disorder (ADD / ADHD) in the second grade, and as a teenager she periodically participated in binge drinking with her friends.

Many years later, when she was 48 years old, Sarah was driving home from work, thinking about her conflicts with her boss. As she neared her neighborhood, she decided to text her friend Jessica to see if she wanted to come over and order pizza. When Sarah looked up from her cell phone and saw the light turn yellow, she pushed harder on the accelerator, but she wasn't quick enough to make it across the intersection. The vehicle coming down the other road caught Sarah's car on its rear bumper. She felt a spinning sensation and then blacked out. Later, she could vaguely recall the paramedics, the leaning telephone pole, and the helicopter ride to the trauma center.

The ER neurologist said Sarah's Glasgow Coma Scale (GCS) score was 14, rating her brain injury as mild. But because she had suffered a brain injury with a seizure as a child, the neurologist ordered a CT scan. The images showed a small area of lost brain tissue called encephalomalacia in the left frontal area. This probably resulted from the old playground injury. There were no other signs of a brain injury, yet months later, Sarah still had persistent symptoms—headache, dizziness, insomnia, and an increase of her usual problems with attention, concentration, and anxiety.

Another former patient, Judy, was 39 years old and had ridden horses for more than twenty years without a serious injury. While she had been thrown off her share of horses over the years, her reliable and steady Ginger had never thrown Judy. Ginger had always smoothly jumped fences, but lately the horse seemed to balk just before a fence. Judy was beginning to admit to herself that her beloved Ginger was aging and growing less agile, but she couldn't bear the thought of giving her up or putting her down. And then it happened. Judy awoke to find her brother leaning over her. She didn't remember how long she had been unaware of her surroundings, but her brother, Jim, guessed it had been about half an hour.

When a concussion occurs at home, family members may transport a person to a hospital's ER or an urgent care center, and that is what Jim did. The family farm was hours from the community hospital. At the ER, Judy's GCS score was a borderline 13, but the CT scan of her head was normal. Because she had a tremor of the left hand and the GCS score was iffy, the physician also ordered an MRI scan. It showed a few tiny hemorrhages in the frontal and temporal lobes, evidence of a Grade I diffuse axonal injury (DAI) (see Chapter 1, Figures 1 and 2). Judy was both distressed to hear this and relieved that no one could tell her she hadn't really had a brain injury, because her symptoms told her something was very wrong.

The American College of Emergency Physicians has set out clear guidelines for concussions to assist with diagnosis, evaluation, and treatment of people 16 years and older with blunt (nonpenetrating) trauma to the brain who come to an ER within twenty-four hours of injury. A physician must first and foremost decide whether to perform a CT scan of the head. A GCS score of 13 to 15 generally suggests a mild brain injury, but because a score of 13 is sometimes associated with poorer outcomes, physicians must take that score more seriously.

In 2004, the World Health Organization Collaborating Centre Task Force, under the leadership of Swedish neuroscientist Jorgen Börg, studied CT scan abnormalities across different severities of

mild brain injury. They found a 5 percent prevalence of patients pre-
senting to a hospital with a GCS of 15 and an abnormal CT. The
number jumped to 30 percent with a GCS score of 13. The term
complicated mild brain injury describes those who have a GCS
score of 13 to 15, but evidence of injury on a CT scan.

Physicians must consider the effects of radiation on patients, especially women of child-bearing age and young children whose
brains are still developing. CT scans are thus typically ordered only
for children who have a history of loss of consciousness, a GCS score
of less than 15, an altered mental status, or clinical evidence of a skull
fracture. A skull fracture is likely if there is blood in the ear canal or
discharge from the ear or nose that might suggest cerebrospinal
fluid. "Raccoon eyes" (blood in the skin around the eyes) or the
"Battle's sign" (blood in the skin behind the ear) are also signs of a
skull fracture.

Just as with adults, certain causes of the injury may also be deciding factors for ordering a CT scan for a child. A fall from three or
more feet or down five or more stairs, a bicycle crash without a
helmet, or a serious motor vehicle crash may indicate a scan is
needed. The red flag rises higher for children 2 years of age or older
who have a history of vomiting after the injury. For the youngest
children, a change in behavior, such as irritability or sleepiness, or
headaches, raises an alarm. And children and adults must be closely
monitored because their condition can deteriorate over time.

Post-Concussion Syndrome Diagnosis

What a patient can expect to experience after a concussion is varied
and often complicated. Post-concussion symptoms overlap with
other conditions such as anxiety, post-traumatic stress disorder
(PTSD), and cervical strain (whiplash). These conditions can be separate from or accompany post-concussion syndrome (PCS). Most

patients with PCS do not have every symptom on the syndrome list. Some patients may have only physical complaints. Others have primarily or exclusively problems with thinking and memory. Still others experience a combination of physical complaints and cognitive, emotional, and behavioral changes. Insomnia and fatigue, both physical and mental, occur frequently after a concussion. Patients vary considerably in terms of the types of symptoms they report, although headaches and dizziness are very common.

The World Health Organization's International Classification of Disease, revision 10 (ICD-10) lists a group of symptoms for PCS: headache, dizziness, fatigue, irritability, difficulty in concentrating and performing mental tasks, memory impairment, insomnia, and reduced tolerance to stress, emotional excitement or alcohol. PCS may also be accompanied by a fear of brain damage, loss of self-esteem, and feelings of depression or anxiety. After Sarah's car accident, the ICD-10 criteria established the diagnosis of PCS. She had severe headaches, dizziness, irritability, and memory problems, and her anxiety had worsened. She also found that she now felt the influence of alcohol after just half a drink. In Judy's case, on the other hand, difficulty concentrating, fatigue, and insomnia were her most prominent symptoms after her fall from the horse.

Many physicians and other providers use symptom checklists to gather data from patients suspected of having a concussion or PCS. These lists can be used to track treatment effectiveness. Harvard surgeon and writer Atul Gawande points out the usefulness of checklists for gathering data and keeping things organized in the chaotic world of medicine in his book *The Checklist Manifesto*. There is evidence, however, that a checklist, or even a very structured interview, may prompt some people to report more symptoms than an open-ended question such as "What is the main symptom you are experiencing?" and then: "What other new symptoms are you experiencing since this happened?" On the other hand, some patients may need prompting to remember various aspects of their recovery.

Basing a diagnosis on a symptom not only means the person must report it, but the test to diagnose the condition must be sensitive and specific. A test is sensitive if it can identify those with the condition (true positives) by ruling out those without it. A test is specific if it is able to identify those without the condition (true negatives) by ruling in those with the condition. Unfortunately, we do not have tests for concussion diagnosis with good sensitivity or specificity.

I have found it essential to screen concussion patients for PTSD given the high rates of exposure to events that trigger acute stress reactions and PTSD (around the time of the concussion or previously during another event). The PC-PTSD, a screening tool developed by Annabelle Prins and colleagues at the National Center for PTSD, US Department of Veterans Affairs, helps for evaluating veterans as well as civilian concussion patients. The first question the PC-PTSD poses is whether the patient has ever been exposed to anything very frightening or horrible, and of course such exposure can happen to anyone in our nation or world today. Examples include a serious accident or fire, physical or sexual assault or abuse, an earthquake or flood, seeing someone killed or seriously injured, having a loved one die through homicide or suicide, or combat experiences.

If the answer to this first question is yes, then the following questions are posed: in the past month, have you: 1) had nightmares about the event or thought about the event when you did not want to? 2) tried hard not to think about the event or went out of your way to avoid situations that reminded you of the event? 3) been constantly on guard, watchful, or easily startled? 4) felt numb or detached from people, activities, or your surroundings? or 5) felt guilty or unable to stop blaming yourself or others for the event or any problems the event may have caused? Answering yes to three out of the five questions suggests probable PTSD.

Limits of Symptom-Based Diagnosis

Symptom-based diagnoses such as we have been discussing can create problems. In one study, neuropsychologist Grant Iverson and his colleagues at Spaulding Rehabilitation Hospital and Harvard Medical School found that close to 8 percent of adults with no concussion history at all experienced enough symptoms to qualify for a diagnosis of PCS. About 15 percent of the group reported moderate to severe symptoms. Iverson and his fellow researchers also became skeptical of symptom-based diagnoses because among a group of student athletes, 19 percent of boys and 28 percent of girls reported symptoms similar to PCS, even though they had not had a recent concussion. Preexisting conditions such as ADD / ADHD, learning disabilities, migraines, psychiatric conditions, and / or a previous concussion were associated with higher rates of PCS symptom reporting.

To further complicate this diagnostic challenge, painful conditions from other injuries can cause symptoms such as fatigue, sleep problems, irritability, and anxiety that can also occur after a concussion. My colleague at Paradigm, physiatrist and senior medical director Steven Moskowitz, makes this important point: "It is always important to remember that not every bump to the head is a concussion, not every memory complaint is a cognitive deficit, and not every headache is a migraine. Patients need a specialist who can decipher unexplained symptoms from a true concussion so that they can provide the most effective care."

Physiatrist Mel Glenn of Spaulding Rehabilitation Hospital and Harvard University emphasizes that in his experience "the causes of post-concussion symptoms vary from person to person and involve an understanding of what happened to the brain, what other areas were injured, pre-injury physical and mental health, and the individual's psychological reaction to the injury." The physician must piece together a mosaic of the individual's personality, life story, and medical and psychosocial history, constructed by sifting through and organizing the patient's own narrative. Here is again why taking a comprehensive history is so crucial.

Sarah's concussions (one in the playground accompanied by a convulsive seizure at age 4, and the other during a car crash at age 48) and her history of ADD / ADHD and substance use made a definitive diagnosis and treatment much more challenging. Sarah's anxiety had been a problem before the car crash, but it worsened. Her headaches and dizziness as well as her intolerance to alcohol appeared only following the accident. (I advised her not to use alcohol, given her substance use history and its potential effects on recovery.) Her story reminds us that no one symptom or set of symptoms alone can fully support a concussion or PCS diagnosis.

Sarah's story is not unusual: a childhood concussion can manifest later in life, and after a second concussion, symptoms and conditions may worsen. Studies show that children who had a concussion before the age of 5 are more likely to show symptoms of ADD / ADHD, conduct disorder, oppositional defiant behavior, substance use disorder, and mood disorder when they reach adolescence. The symptoms and signs of these conditions can overlap with those of a brain injury, so concussions in very young children may go unrecognized. Megan Narad and her colleagues at Cincinnati Children's Hospital Medical Center found in their research that very young children were almost four times more likely than control subjects to develop secondary ADHD after TBI (even mild TBI or concussion). They followed patients for up to ten years; on average, attentional problems developed about seven years after the TBI.

Circumstances for workers may pose additional challenges. Workers' compensation provides medical benefits and wage replacement for employees injured while at work. The tradeoff is that the employee forfeits the right to sue his or her employer in exchange for receiving disability benefits and health care (and, if death occurs, life insurance) for any condition related to the work injury. Payments for pain and suffering or for employer negligence are not usually part of the deal. In some cases, workers fear retaliation from their employers if they file a workers' compensation claim, a reason they may not report injuries or pursue company grievance processes or litigation.

Some workers may show poor effort, exaggerate or magnify symptoms, or even malinger (feign symptoms or problems). However, as New York psychiatrist Jonathan Silver points out, other unconscious factors such as stereotype threat may operate in these cases. Stereotype threat is society's bias against a subgroup—such as an ethnic or sexual minority, or a person with a cognitive disability—as perceived by a member of the subgroup. Silver states, "The observation that expectation predicts prognosis . . . emphasizes that there are many aspects to symptom production. While anxiety may impair performance, expectations about the prognosis of brain injury, either initially or through stereotype threat, may increase symptoms."

My patient Pablo, a construction worker who fell from scaffolding, had not finished high school in Mexico because of his family's economic situation and the consequent need to work when he was only 15. He immigrated to the United States at age 20 to work in construction. He underwent a neuropsychological evaluation about three months after his injury. Because he was unfamiliar with the kind of testing the neuropsychologist gave him, his anxiety was intense when he took the tests. The testing showed that he likely had not achieved an expected level of education beyond grade 8, and he had some problems associated with the concussion, namely attention and memory deficits. The neuropsychologist took all of this into account in the interpretation of the results. Repeat testing after more recovery at six months was less stressful for him. His story continues in Chapters 3 and 9.

Assessing Athletes

Athletes present a different set of diagnostic challenges than workers and other people with a history of concussion. As a group, athletes are highly motivated and used to participating in sports intensely, even with pain and discomfort, so they are often hesitant to come forward with symptoms. Athletes may also deny or underreport their symptoms because they don't want to jeopardize their shot at a scholarship or a position on a team, or because they simply want to get back in the game. Sadly, they may not fully understand the injury's seriousness. Children and youth may not be aware of their symptoms or of the meaning of symptoms they experience after a concussion. Boys and men playing team sports may be less likely than girls and women to report symptoms. Athletes also fear that they may be forbidden to play a sport that forms a big part of their identities and social worlds and has the potential to provide substantial financial rewards.

A fear of being removed from play perennially recurs in sports-related concussion news. New England Patriots quarterback Tom Brady, for example, made news when he contradicted his wife's account of his 2017 concussions. She said he had had several; he said he didn't have any. Professional athletes certainly have career reasons for not reporting symptoms, but they are not the only ones who fail to report their injuries.

Michael McCrea and colleagues found that 15 percent of high school football players across twenty schools in Milwaukee, Wisconsin, reported a concussion during the 2002 football season. Nearly 30 percent reported a previous history of concussion. But among the athletes who responded to the survey, more than 40 percent of those who had suffered a concussion said they had knowingly hid their symptoms in order to stay in a game. One out of five athletes in the survey group indicated that they would be unlikely or very unlikely to report concussion symptoms to a coach or athletic trainer. Among these players' most common reasons for not reporting a concussion: they did not think the injury was serious enough, did not want to be withheld from competition, or lacked awareness that their symptoms resulted from the concussion they had sustained.

Daniel Torres and colleagues published results from a similar survey ten years later and also found that more than 40 percent of those with a history of concussion disclosed that they had knowingly hidden symptoms of a concussion in order to stay in a game. Twenty-two percent of the athletes surveyed indicated that they would be unlikely or very unlikely to report concussion symptoms to a coach or athletic trainer in the future. Ironically, the majority also said they had received education about concussion.

Concussions acquired on the athletic field cause similar symptoms to those injuries incurred off the field. There are, however, important differences. A person injured in a fall, an assault, or a motor vehicle crash is more likely than a young athlete to be taken out of harm's way, so nonathletes are far less likely to suffer a second concussion than athletes. In most cases of sports concussion, a trainer or coach evaluates athletes at the scene, and then a physician or licensed health-care provider sees them in an outpatient office or ER.

Most guidelines now require that an athlete must not return to play on the same day that the concussion occurred and should not return to play until a physician or other licensed health professional has cleared them to do so.

Since nine out of ten sports concussions occur without a loss of consciousness, and many happen without a direct hit to the head, the signs of a significant injury to the brain can be subtle. Diagnosing a concussion is also more difficult when symptoms do not fully emerge until days after the initial injury. The term "subconcussion" refers to an injury to the brain in the absence of immediate symptoms or signs (or ones so fleeting that no one knows the brain has been injured). Diagnosis of a subconcussion occurs after the fact, as delayed symptoms emerge, or if an imaging study shows evidence of brain injury. It's a term that reminds us again of the challenges of a symptom-based diagnosis.

In most cases of concussion, athletes become confused and disoriented. They may experience memory difficulties, double vision, headaches, dizziness, or balance problems in the immediate aftermath. The description of a concussion from a javelin injury in the ancient Greek epic *The Iliad* resembles, albeit in more flowery language, what we see on sports television and in real-time high school and college athletics:

> Without a wound the Trojan hero stands;
> But yet so stunn'd that, staggering on the plain,
> His arm and knee his sinking bulk sustain;
> O'er his dim sight the misty vapours rise,
> And a short darkness shades his swimming eyes.

Epidemiologist Nancy Carney and her co-authors analyzed the medical literature to identify the most common features of concussions diagnosed on the basis of observation and those features that might predict whether or not a concussion had actually occurred. They concluded that disorientation or confusion occurs immediately after the injury, followed by impaired balance at the time of the incident or within one day. Within 48 hours of a concussion, other problems such as slower reaction time or impaired learning and memory may emerge. This delay in emergence of difficulties may be due to the cascade of cellular events described in Chapter 1, or simply because daily life presents more cognitive challenges as time passes.

Carla and Tom

The stories of former patients of mine, Carla and Tom, demonstrate the diagnosis problem particular to sports concussions. At age 17, when she was a junior in high school, Carla had her first concussion when she collided with another player during soccer practice. Although she staggered to the sidelines, she did not tell anyone about her headaches, dizziness, memory problems, and difficulty focusing. She returned to practice the next day. At a game a few days later, she headed a ball, collided with another player, and then fell, hitting her head on the turf.

When I examined Carla six weeks later, her recovery seemed to have stalled. She still experienced headaches, dizziness, insomnia, and difficulty concentrating in class. She could scarcely remember if she had completed her homework. She and her parents were very worried about the continuation and progression of her symptoms. Would she lose her chance at a college scholarship? Her parents were eager for me to declare her fit to start playing again. Carla's father was also her soccer coach. His other players with concussions had recovered quickly and fully, with a few successfully winning college athletic scholarships. He had high hopes that Carla would win one, too.

Tom, a college football defensive end, was 22 years old when he encountered a deer crossing an icy country road as he drove through rural Pennsylvania in the 1980s, before airbags were common. Tom's head cracked the windshield, and he briefly lost consciousness. At the local hospital ER, he was confused and moved unsteadily. The CT brain scan showed no evidence of a brain injury. The hospital sent him home with a requirement that he be supervised 24 / 7, instructing him and his family to watch for vomiting or changes in his level of consciousness, but recommending no other treatment.

As the days and weeks passed, it became clear to Tom's parents that their son had serious problems. He couldn't remember where he went to college. In fact, in some cases, he couldn't remember his high school friends' names or much about them. Tom had had multiple concussions playing football as a child and adolescent, as well as a few concussions during high school practices. His mother wondered during Tom's first appointment with me whether these sports concussions related to his difficulties after the car accident. Was his football career, or even his college career, over?

Young athletes like Carla and Tom have a lot at stake. Many participate in sports because of the camaraderie, the chance to excel, and the sheer enjoyment of the sport itself. Their identities, self-worth, and social communities are tied to their participation in team sports. The sports culture pushes them toward achievement, and toward putting up with pain and angst. These factors complicate the diagnosis and management of concussion in athletes.

Primary and Specialty Care

Researcher Kristy Arbogast and her colleagues at the Children's Hospital of Philadelphia found that only about 20 percent of children with concussions were seen in ERs in a regional health system, and this is likely the case in many parts of the United States. Pediatricians or other primary care physicians are the most likely to evaluate children with suspected concussions. The less-chaotic primary care clinic in fact may be a better setting than the ER for in-depth interviewing and more careful examination to fully determine exposure to a concussive event and the post-concussion symptoms that may arise. However, in all cases, concussions must be viewed as serious events that require urgent or even emergency assessment.

Expertise, examination skills, and available clinic time in different medical specialties vary widely among physicians and other health-care providers. Primary care physicians see a variety of patients with challenging conditions, but for ongoing management, many prefer to triage patients to concussion clinics or rehabilitation centers better organized to deal with the complexity of post-concussion symptoms. More and more concussion clinics are opening to meet increasing demand, especially for diagnosis and treatment of sports concussions. These clinics usually use a team approach, as do rehabilitation facilities serving patients with concussions. They employ health-care professionals with a range of specialties to provide their expertise and assemble pieces of the puzzle. The best care for patients with unresolved symptoms occurs in these settings, where clinicians can easily communicate with each other and provide team-based care.

People with concussions need more than just acute care evaluation and management, however. They also want and need education about what to expect during the recovery process and estimates about how the recovery timeframe will unfold. Without education, patients do not understand what is happening to them, and they may catastrophize (think the worst can happen) or develop anxiety or depression. Most concussions follow a typical progression toward recovery. First, the person experiences a range of acute symptoms that worsen if they try to resume activities too quickly. Certain activities, such as using computers, reading, or exercising intensely, may exacerbate some symptoms. With proper treatment and education, symptoms gradually resolve for most people, and recovery usually progresses over weeks or months. If symptoms do not resolve by three months, comprehensive neuropsychological testing can be very helpful to guide further treatment decisions.

Neuropsychological Evaluation

The evaluation of cognitive functioning in people with TBIs, or neuropsychological evaluations, has benefited from major recent advances in medicine. Neuropsychologists, the psychologists who administer and interpret the tests that form part of these evaluations, have extensive training in brain anatomy, brain function, and the consequences of brain injury or disease. A neuropsychologist can help answer questions about whether a significant brain injury has occurred and whether residual effects remain from the injury, because certain patterns of deficits occur after TBI and concussions.

A neuropsychological evaluation typically involves an interview with the patient, family, and significant others. Following the interviews, a neuropsychologist usually administers paper and pencil testing in a structured environment. The purpose of the interview is to glean information about how the person functions in an unstructured, more complex, and distracting environment than that imposed by test-taking.

Neuropsychologists use batteries of standardized tests to determine levels of cognitive function in specific domains such as attention, memory, reasoning, language function, problem-solving, information processing speed, verbal ability and verbal memory, visual-spatial ability and visual memory, personality, and symptom validity. The neuropsychologist also evaluates academic skills and emotional functioning. Neuropsychological testing can provide information about the degree of patient effort, motivation, or even malingering (feigning symptoms or problems).

There is no clear consensus on the test battery to use for a patient with a concussion or concussion-related symptoms or signs. Determining pre-injury levels of cognitive function is difficult, but this can be estimated using previous levels of achievement in education or employment or by requesting standardized testing from school records for comparison. Neuropsychological testing takes about six hours. A shorter battery of tests can be administered early in the course of recovery, and a full evaluation can be deferred until painful conditions have been treated effectively and any psychological conditions stabilized. Some recovery or complete recovery usually occurs, especially with milder injuries, so improvement in deficit areas can also help make the diagnosis if repeat testing is given six months to a year after the first evaluation.

Northern California clinical neuropsychologist Ernest Bryant explained his point of view to me regarding the testing he does in his practice: "Cognitive deficits can be subtle, and affective symptoms like depression, anxiety, and irritability can arise from multiple causes. In addition to a detailed interview and medical record review, comprehensive neuropsychological testing should incorporate testing directed at teasing out which are (and are not) true post-concussion symptoms. The results of the evaluation can help determine, for example, if a student should have extra time for test-taking, an athlete should retire from a sport, or a worker can start back to work part-time. There may be evidence of pre-existing psychological issues that have worsened, and litigation may be a factor in these complex evaluations, so they should be performed by a board-certified clinical neuropsychologist." For patients with prolonged post-concussion symptoms who are disabled in relation to work, school, or other activities, a clinical neuropsychologist can help with both diagnosis and treatment planning.

The NCATs

Neurocognitive assessment tests (NCATs) are paper-and-pencil or computer-based tools that are used to determine the likelihood of a concussion or more severe TBI—whether on the battlefield or the athletic field. An NCAT can assist in diagnosis only if it can accurately measure the domains of functioning it purports to measure, and if it produces consistent results. NCATs have not undergone the extensive research that establishes their sensitivity or specificity (ruling a concussion in or out), validity (accuracy of measurement), and reliability (repeatability) of older neuropsychological test batteries. In some cases, test developers, not independent researchers, have conducted the research, and conflicts of interest may interfere with results.

The results of different NCATs can't really be compared, because each differs slightly in terms of test items, computer-user interfaces, scoring, and methods of analysis. The sports world and the military have been developing and using NCATs for several decades. (See Chapter 9 for discussion of the military.) NCATs measure performance at a given point in time, but they do not directly assess brain structure or function, and many factors can influence the results of these tests. These instruments serve primarily as screening tools, and as such, they are insufficient for diagnosing a brain injury.

Carla's Early Evaluations

A coach (an assistant coach, not her father) evaluated Carla on the sidelines after her concussion. The coach used an NCAT called the Sports Concussion Assessment Test (SCAT). The SCAT includes the Standardized Assessment of Concussion (SAC), the Graded Symptom Checklist, and sideline questions. Although its scientific validity and reliability are limited, the SCAT can be used to assess athletes with suspected concussions in the minutes and hours following injury. Carla's results were concerning enough for the coach to decide to take her off the field. Carla reported a severe headache and dizziness, her balance seemed off, and she couldn't answer all the sideline questions correctly, including the one about last week's game: "Who was the opposing team?"

Carla still suffered from severe headaches and dizziness three weeks after the second concussion. She wasn't sleeping more than four hours a night. Her primary care physician rightly said she didn't need a CT scan because she scored a perfect 15 on the Glasgow Coma Scale and performed normally on a standard neurological exam, including tests of balance. Carla's school had administered an NCAT called the ImPACT (Immediate Post-Concussion Assessment and Cognitive Testing) on all its athletes at the beginning of the school year, and Carla's results were available as a baseline. Her scores when she took the test again confirmed she was having new difficulty in verbal memory, processing speed, and reaction time.

Schools and the sports industry sometimes administer NCATs for baseline testing of groups of athletes. Theoretically, comparison of scores on pre-injury and post-injury tests of cognitive abilities might be a valid means to determine if concussion-related impairments are present. However, promoting these computerized instruments as baseline tests may need a check. Indianapolis Colts quarterback Peyton Manning admitted that he intentionally tried to "sandbag" (underperform) on the National Football League's preseason baseline concussion test so he could remain off the injury report if he suffered a concussion during the season. Younger athletes may do the same. Return-to-play decisions are being made based on test scores, and athletes who want to keep playing try to game the system.

In 2016, the US Food and Drug Administration (FDA) approved the marketing of the ImPACT (and its pediatric version for children ages 5 to 11) as a medical device for assessing cognitive function following a possible concussion. The ImPACT software runs on a desktop or laptop, and a licensed health professional—a physician, neuropsychologist, or speech therapist—can perform and interpret the results with training. The ImPACT tests the cognitive functions of verbal and visual memory, reaction time, processing speed, and word recognition. Clinicians can compare the results to age-matched controls.

Medical device companies have aggressively marketed various other screening devices that then make the mainstream news. Among the array of devices that have arrived on the market are helmet and mouth-guard sensors that measure impact on the athletic field; virtual reality headsets; eye-tracking software; video equipment; smartphone apps that screen reaction of the pupils; quantitative EEG monitors; and an apparatus that measures responses to sound and pitch. Given the numbers of people with concussions and increasing attention to the problem of diagnosis, the list of these devices will no doubt grow. The public should view all of these devices as potentially useful but be cognizant of whether research backs up the promises.

The FDA has warned manufacturers not to market, and the public not to use, medical devices that claim to help assess, diagnose, or manage TBI, including concussions, that the FDA has not approved. Even those FDA-approved devices such as the ImPACT require an evaluation by a physician or other licensed health-care provider. In any case, these devices will always remain adjuncts to diagnosis behind the critically important history-taking and physical examination that only a physician or other qualified health-care professional can provide.

Carla's Later Evaluations

Carla's primary care physician referred her to my outpatient concussion clinic at a rehabilitation center. The Montreal Cognitive Assessment (MoCA), a brief screen of her cognitive function, showed that she had problems with attention and memory, although distractions from a headache or just plain stress could have affected the results. She was retested using a different version of the MoCA at follow-up appointments, and her scores improved. There remained a question about whether her improvement in subsequent testing was due to the "practice effect." Did the repeated experience of being asked the same or similar questions help her do better? She needed a neuropsychological evaluation to more accurately define the cognitive problems she was having.

Carla underwent testing using tools that measure the complex networks described in Chapter 1 (see Figure 6), including the Balance Error Scoring System (BESS) to test her balance and a computerized version of the King-Devick (KD) test to evaluate her eye movements. The KD is a flashcard system first used by schools in the late 1970s to help detect eye movement disorders in children with learning disabilities, and it is now widely used as a sideline or outpatient concussion screening tool.

Carla also underwent a vestibular / ocular motor screening (VOMS) assessment to measure eye movements such as smooth pursuits (visual tracking), saccades (quick movements of the eyes between fixation points), near point of convergence (distance the eyes are both able to move inward toward an approaching object), and the vestibular ocular reflex (VOR). The VOR triggers the eyes to move in the opposite direction when the head is moved. In other words, the VOR coordinates eye movement with head movement, enabling us to see clearly and maintain balance as we move around. Disruption or damage in the VOR can cause movement-related dizziness, nausea, blurred vision, and difficulty maintaining balance when the head moves. Carla's symptoms worsened with these tests. She had a lot of difficulty with balance on the BESS also.

Based on the results of these evaluations, Carla was evaluated by a neuro-optometrist, a vestibular physical therapist, and a speech and language pathologist. Because she continued to have cognitive symptoms and difficulties when she returned to school, she underwent a comprehensive neuropsychological evaluation. The tests included the Wechsler Adult Intelligence Scale, the California Verbal Learning Test to assess her memory, the Wisconsin Card Sorting Test to evaluate her executive functions, the Rey-Osterrieth Complex Figure to test her visual-perceptual skills and visual memory abilities, and other tests, administered over about six hours. She showed problems in verbal but not visual memory, and impairments in executive functions such as complex attention, mental flexibility, and organizational skills. These results helped her high school to provide classroom and other accommodations (see Chapter 3).

The Patient's Voice

We still don't have sophisticated or universally accepted methods to diagnose a concussion or to link symptoms to brain networks. An age-old disregard for concussion's importance, a lack of research funding, and the complexity inherent in the disorder all contribute to this frustrating situation. The advanced neuroimaging and laboratory biomarkers described in Chapter 1 will eventually become available for routine testing in patients with concussions. Better tools for evaluating cognitive, visual, and vestibular systems will also become available. Other technologies will help with diagnosing psychiatric disorders such as PTSD, anxiety, or depression, and chronic pain conditions such as the headaches that often accompany these injuries. These advances will expand our current capabilities to offer patients scientific treatment and more accurate predictions of their recovery timeframes.

Systems scientist Erin Kenzie and her associates in Oregon and Utah make a good case for concussion as a complex disease that requires a comprehensive approach. This approach must take into account the injury and its scientific aspects as well as the concussed person's unique experiences. During several interviews, Seth Fischer, a medical student who experienced a concussion in a bicycle accident during medical school, spoke to me about the complexity of his injury, its aftermath, and his concern about the unmet needs of patients with chronic post-concussion symptoms:

> The convoluted nature of these injuries is one thing that our profession doesn't understand and one thing that is really hard for the patient to elaborate on. I didn't know what was going on. I learned a lot about how to listen to patients. The chronic nature of injuries, whether it's memory problems or headaches, is a terrible existence. It's something that doesn't go away. [A physician] might see the patient once every couple of weeks or months and see them progressing. For the patient, it's a slow slog. It's hard to make people understand this. With a brain injury it's a whole different game. It's a slow trajectory.

Dr. Fischer is training to be an anesthesiologist. He urges physicians and other health-care providers to take concussion and its consequences seriously.

More than fifty years ago, neurosurgeon Alex Taylor recognized the same challenges medical professionals and patients face today when he wrote in the *British Medical Journal:* "That a patient should complain of organically determined symptoms of headache, dizziness, lack of energy, poor memory, and difficulty in concentrating and have no physical signs is to some doctors incredible. But the central nervous system is unique in its clinical silence." Taylor clearly gave patients with post-concussion symptoms the benefit of the doubt. He understood that the concussed brain is a mystery because science cannot yet completely explain a patient's symptoms in terms of brain pathways. Medicine is indeed an imperfect science.

We need to measure a patient's symptoms and suffering with science and technology where we can, but technology will never be able to describe a patient's experience. Physicians can come close to understanding the patient experience only by listening and probing, activities that require time and attention. Even if concussion-detection technology advances, concussion diagnosis and treatment will remain complicated. Some patients will not have a smooth, fast, or even complete recovery. But successful treatment, the subject of the next chapter, is only possible if physicians first listen carefully, and always avoid a dismissive diagnosis.

3

Concussion Care

IN CHAPTER 12 of *Persuasion,* Jane Austen's last completed novel, published posthumously in 1818, Louisa Musgrove falls and suffers a concussion. Her then suitor Captain Wentworth fails to persuade her not to run and jump into his arms: He "thought the jar too great; but no, he reasoned and talked in vain, she smiled and said, 'I am determined I will:' he put out his hands; she was too precipitate by half a second, she fell on the pavement on the Lower Cobb, and was taken up lifeless!"

Austen does not trivialize the event: "As to the sad catastrophe itself . . . it was perfectly decided that it had been the consequence of much thoughtlessness and much imprudence; that its effects were most alarming, and that it was frightful to think, how long Miss Musgrove's recovery might yet be doubtful, and how liable she would still remain to suffer from the concussion hereafter!" A physician, conveniently nearby, administers smelling salts, and Louisa recovers consciousness within a short period of time, although probably not because of the salts. Her sister-in-law, Mary, remains with her during her recovery, which occupies much of the rest of the novel.

One wonders if Austen had personal knowledge about concussion as a possibly serious medical event without a clear prognosis. Ten chapters later, Louisa's recovery remains incomplete. Louisa has "very much recovered," although she is "altered" in the months following her fall. Louisa's new suitor, Captain Benwick, is attentive, but it isn't clear that Louisa received any treatment other than rest: "there is no running or jumping about, no laughing or dancing; it is quite different. If one happens only to shut the door a little hard, she starts and wriggles like a young dab-chick in the water; and Benwick sits at her elbow, reading verses, or whispering to her, all day long." Two centuries later, prescriptions for rest versus activity, a treatment dilemma raised in Louisa's story, remain a focus of debate in post-concussion care and treatment.

Acute Care

Just as Jane Austen wrote in *Persuasion,* when a concussion occurs, medical care should be sought immediately. The most important thing anyone should do after a concussion (or a suspected concussion) is to stop activity and seek medical help. A call to a primary care physician's office can sometimes result in a same-day appointment. However, evaluation at the closest emergency room (ER) or urgent care center is prudent. A prompt evaluation is important to assess the severity of the concussion and to determine if there are any signs that the injury will progress.

Severe vomiting, seizures, deepening sleep, new numbness, weakness, balance problems, double vision, difference in the size or shape of the pupils, eye pain, vision loss, or severe headaches may signal a progressive problem in the brain or the eye. Sometimes, a hidden problem such as a malformation in the brain that has not before been associated with symptoms becomes more obvious. For example, an Arnold–Chiari I (ACM) malformation can go unnoticed until headaches, dizziness, weakness or numbness of the arms, incoordination, or other symptoms occur after a concussion. This rare congenital abnormality occurs during fetal development; the cerebellum at the back of the brain protrudes slightly into the foramen magnum (the opening in the skull at the bottom of the head). Neurosurgeon Michael Wan and his University of Toronto colleagues conducted a chart review to look for patients who had no ACM symptoms before but acquired symptoms after trauma. They concluded that minor head or neck trauma can precipitate symptoms suggestive of concussion or whiplash in patients with a previously undiagnosed ACM.

A medical emergency may occur after a concussion, especially in the elderly, or an emergency can evolve over minutes, hours, or days. For example, Barbara, an older woman who hit her head when she fell in her bathroom, experienced progressive physical and mental impairments over twenty-four hours because of delayed bleeding in her brain. (See Chapter 8 for more on this kind of injury.) The unfortunate reality is that we don't really have good ways to measure concussion severity at the time the injury happens, nor can we perfectly predict what may happen over time. Fortunately, dire outcomes are rare.

Treatments for concussion and post-concussion symptoms have certainly advanced since Austen's time, but many people still have difficulty finding and paying for specialized concussion care, starting with expert diagnosis and followed by targeted treatments. Emergency medical systems, insurance coverage, and variations in health-system staffing affect how people access care in the United States and around the world. Diagnosis rates vary widely across geographic areas due to variations in incidence, availability of care, practice patterns, or database coding protocols.

Aside from determining concussion severity, an initial treatment goal is to educate patients and families. For more than two decades, we know that early education and reassurance from concussion experts is the key for improving outcomes, especially for post-concussion symptoms. Australian neuroscience researcher Jennie Ponsford demonstrated the effectiveness of early education in patients with concussion in a 2002 study. Simply giving patients a booklet with information and coping strategies one week after an injury appeared to help decrease symptoms at three months in her study. Too much information can be overwhelming, but physicians and other health-care providers can answer additional questions and give reassurance at follow-up appointments.

Early treatment and education can prevent chronic, intractable problems from developing. The good news is that a comprehensive treatment program targeting symptoms, and adequate follow-up care, can result in excellent outcomes for people who have had a concussion.

Follow-Up Care

Ideally, ongoing concussion care should take place in settings staffed with physicians such as physiatrists or neurologists, and other providers with the expertise to treat concussions and other traumatic injuries and psychological conditions. Broad-based concussion clinics treat injured athletes and also people with workplace injuries, veterans, the young, and the elderly. A developing child, adolescent, and elderly person respond to a concussion with different patterns and timing of recovery. Children and young adolescents with concussions should be treated by physicians trained in pediatric medical care. These might be pediatricians, pediatric neurologists, or pediatric physiatrists.

A concussion clinic physician may be board-certified in the newer medical specialty of brain injury medicine (BIM). This sub-specialty certification is available to physicians with primary specialization in PM&R (physiatry), neurology (including child neurology), and psychiatry. Rehabilitation outpatient departments in adult or pediatric centers offer an ideal setting for evaluating patients of all ages with concussion. Physiatrists typically staff these departments, and some physiatrists have additional certification or experience in BIM, pediatric rehabilitation, sports medicine, or pain management. These physicians collaborate with other rehabilitation providers such as neuropsychologists, physical therapists, occupational therapists, speech and language pathologists, neuro-ophthalmologists, neuro-optometrists, rehabilitation nurses, and social workers. An interdisciplinary team with this range of expertise can evaluate and treat post-concussion symptoms, associated chronic pain, other injuries, and psychological conditions. Not all patients need all or even most of these services. However, for those who do, the benefits are clear.

Physiatrists and other rehabilitation providers typically use a biopsychosocial model for treating post-concussion symptoms and conditions involving pain. Internist and psychiatrist George Engel originated this model of care delivery in the 1960s. Engel believed that to fully understand and respond to a patient's suffering, clinicians must address the biological, psychological, and social dimensions of their illness as well as their physical symptoms. Engel described his model as an alternative to both the biomedical model of industrialized societies and to the Freudian psychoanalytic model. In the 1970s and 1980s, the biopsychosocial model promoted the development of interdisciplinary care, exemplified in certain fields of medicine such as psychiatry, PM&R, and other rehabilitation fields. The American Academy of Physical Medicine and Rehabilitation offers listings of physiatrists with subspecialties in brain injury medicine, sports medicine, or pain medicine on its website.

Sports medicine physicians have extensive experience treating athletes with injuries, including concussions. Sports medicine is a subspecialty of medicine, and board certification is available to orthopedists, physiatrists, and primary care specialists. Physicians and other professionals with expertise in many different sports-related injuries staff sports medicine clinics and provide expert and comprehensive care for athletes. However, sports medicine physicians and their clinic staff most often treat injuries to muscles, bones, and joints. The services and programs sports concussion clinics offer also vary, because there is so far little standardization of practices or accreditation, and many clinics treat only athletes. The Boston-based Concussion Legacy Foundation has tips and resources to help people find reputable sports concussion clinics.

Rest or Exercise?

In the nineteenth and twentieth centuries, doctors recommended rest for anyone with a concussion. Sometimes that included bedrest or sedentary activities within the home, as in Louisa Musgrove's case. In the twenty-first century, the concussion literature still uses varying definitions of rest. A practical definition of physical rest makes a distinction between the absence of athletic activities on the one hand, and daily activities that require exertion on the other. Sitting out football practice doesn't mean you can't go grocery shopping, mow the lawn, or lift free weights at the gym. Cognitive rest, on the other hand, refers to minimizing high-concentration activities that exacerbate concussion symptoms, such as computer use, reading and writing, and watching television. For people with concussion symptoms, these activities may be challenges at home or school, in the community, or at work.

After a concussion, biochemical events alter cerebral blood flow, cellular metabolism, and cellular structures during a period of vulnerability. This vulnerable period is the basis for current guidelines requiring removal from play and protection from another concussion or second impact syndrome. Re-exposing the developing brains of children, adolescents, and young adults during this vulnerable period can cause further damage. Return-to-play decisions are a complicated matter because imaging studies suggest that using symptoms to determine return to risky activities is itself risky because brain abnormalities persist after symptoms resolve (see Chapters 1 and 6).

Very intense exercise shortly following an injury may cause harm because exercise compels higher metabolic demands on the body. Cerebral blood flow and glucose metabolism differ in children and adolescents. The reality is that scientists don't yet have complete answers about when a person who has had a brain injury can safely resume exercise, or what kinds of exercise are safe. But some clinical research suggests that activity, even light exercise, might be the best medicine after a concussion. Total rest beyond a day, and even relative rest beyond a few days, can prolong symptoms.

The brain may not respond well to inactivity. Low-level exercise may actually hasten recovery or even improve it. We know that exercise can effectively treat anxiety, depression, and mood regulation, and that bedrest can contribute to poorer recoveries and disability after injury or illness. We also know from studies of more severe TBIs that exercise promotes brain-derived neurotrophic factor (BDNF), which stimulates the growth of neural stem cells and new synapses, a process called neurogenesis.

Differing statements by the authors of the International Conferences' Consensus Statements in the last two conferences—Zurich in

2013 and Berlin in 2017—reflect a shift in thinking among clinicians about post-concussion rest. The Zurich group recommended physical and cognitive rest until symptoms resolve. The Berlin group's statement shows the shift: "After a brief period of initial rest (24–48 hours), symptom-limited activity can be begun while staying below a cognitive and physical exacerbation threshold." This newer recommendation limits the period of rest and encourages earlier activity. In 2018, the American Academy of Pediatrics also revised its 2010 mild TBI guideline, changing the period of rest to no more than two to three days. Unfortunately, for some individuals, especially young people, 24 to 48 hours may be too short a period for enough symptom resolution. The science of concussion is still primarily based on consensus rather than solid research evidence, and this serves as another example of the imperfect science of medicine.

After a concussion, patients may need to take some time away from work or school to decrease stressful contributions to their symptoms, but they should continue activities outside the home. A return to normal activities (including work or school) should occur as soon as a patient can tolerate them. When a person returns to mental or physical activity after a concussion, the key is to start slowly. An assistive device such as a cane or a shower chair can aid balance and coordination in the days, weeks, or months after a concussion, especially for older people. Certain activities, such as aerobic exercise, may make symptoms worse, but frequent breaks or a reduction in the intensity of the activity can help. A patient may need to minimize time reading or looking at a screen if these activities bring on or intensify symptoms such as headaches.

Concussion may affect a patient's reaction time and the ability to alternate visual attention, both of which are critical for driving. Patients should discuss driving with their physicians, who may advise against it during the recovery period after a concussion. A physician may refer a patient they suspect is not capable of driving for a certified driver evaluation (usually conducted by an occupational therapist).

Carla's Treatment

My patient Carla, the high school soccer player introduced in Chapter 2, had a high resting heart rate, and she startled easily. Her heart rate and blood pressure showed little variability with exercise compared with rest, a sign that there might be a disturbance to her autonomic nervous system associated with her concussions. Treadmill exercise helped her to improve her aerobic skills, and gradually her heart rate and blood pressure readings began to vary in a normal way. The program began with light aerobic exercise during which she did not have symptoms, so over time she progressed to moderate to intense exercise. Her symptoms did not re-emerge during this progression.

Primary care sports medicine physician John Leddy and his team in Buffalo, New York, research exercise as a treatment for concussion. They developed the Buffalo Concussion Treadmill Test to help determine when athletes are ready to return to their sport. The protocol works for nonathletes, too. The Buffalo researchers distinguish between different subgroups of people with concussion. For example, they parse out those with neck-related headaches, migraine headaches, visual or vestibular (equilibrium and balance) problems, and those with blood pressure and heart rate differences.

The Treadmill Test can be used to design a home exercise program with a maximum heart rate protocol for patients with post-concussion symptoms. The exercise protocols that Leddy and his group utilize are controlled and graded (sequenced) exercises, and provide an exercise prescription unique for a person, given his or her symptoms, physical examination, medical conditions, and other factors that might determine best outcomes. A physician or physical therapist must guide the program.

Carla returned to classes and resumed academic work through a return-to-learn program. She required some accommodations, such as extra time for test-taking and homework, until about seven months after her second concussion. Finally, she participated in sport-specific and noncontact athletic training before starting back to workouts in soccer practices. She resumed playing in games a year after her second concussion, and received a soccer scholarship to attend the college of her choice.

Symptom-Based Care

A symptom checklist completed by the patient, or symptom information otherwise gathered, can help identify which symptoms require treatment. Physicians can also use this to chart what changes happen over time during treatment. Frequent follow-up is necessary in the months after a concussion, especially if a patient experiences debilitating symptoms. Re-evaluation of symptoms and repeat medical examinations should always continue until symptoms resolve.

Concussion symptoms fall into three categories: physical, mood- and sleep-related, and cognitive. Relationships among concussion symptoms often make treatment challenging. For example, pain can affect sleep, attention, and mood. Sleep deprivation can affect mood, make painful conditions worse, and cause cognitive problems. Cognitive problems can produce anxiety, and then anxiety leads to sleep problems. The best outcomes are achieved when people receive information and therapeutic interventions soon after their injury. Later, problems and symptoms may be compounded by the stress of illness and fear of the unknown.

Mel Glenn, physiatrist at Harvard's Spaulding Rehabilitation Center, sees education about the compounding effects of anxiety as key: "Education about how the effects of anxiety's contribution to making symptoms worse can actually help to alleviate the anxiety." He also pointed out that some people may have a tendency to think that their symptoms are new, when in fact they may not be new. Some clinicians have referred to this as "the good old days" syndrome. For example, Sarah, my patient who was injured during childhood and was later involved in a car crash, had generalized anxiety before her injury that she sometimes tried to relieve with alcohol. When her primary care physician strongly recommended that she had to give up alcohol, she became more anxious, which she attributed to her newly diagnosed concussion (see Chapter 2).

While it would be great if a pill could magically cure a concussion, medications are not the primary treatment for concussion and post-concussion symptoms. Rehabilitation strategies such as educating patients and families about concussion and its effects, regularizing sleep-wake cycles, and prescribing an individualized exercise program often offer more help than medication. Treatment targets specific symptoms such as headaches, dizziness and vertigo, and cognitive difficulties.

Complementary or alternative medicine treatment refers to methods outside the mainstream conventions. These lack strong evidence for effectiveness but may be helpful for some people after a concussion. Veterans Health Administration physiatrist David Cifu uses an integrative medicine approach for veterans with brain injuries, including concussions, with "the full palette of safe and potentially efficacious interventions, used judiciously and blended (or integrated) to meet the needs of each individual." He states that with an integrative approach, "there is no need to label treatments as Western, Eastern, alternative, or otherwise." Acupuncture or tai chi, for example, can be very helpful interventions for some individuals with acute and chronic pain, decreasing the need for medications. Other nondrug approaches, such as mindfulness and biofeedback, can help some people who are experiencing post-concussion symptoms.

The unfortunate reality is that very few treatments for concussion, even conventional treatments, have strong scientific evidence supporting their efficacy. That said, turning to unconventional treatments not covered by insurance may be costly. It is always best to seek advice and referrals from a physician who has completed a thorough evaluation and can assess the potential benefits and risks of unconventional care.

Sleep and the Brain

The Centers for Disease Control and Prevention (CDC) reports that many Americans are sleep-deprived. In the 1980s, the number was about one-quarter of Americans. Forty years later, almost one-third of us do not get enough sleep. Adults need an average of seven to eight hours of sleep per night, and teens require eight to ten hours, although requirements vary from person to person. Most important is a stable sleep pattern. Sleep contributes to immune function, memory, mental health and fatigue prevention, and maybe even longevity.

Sleep disruptions can affect concussion recovery because they affect the body's normal processes of restoration during sleep. Scientists are exploring the brain's inflammatory system to shed light on how concussions might produce the symptoms and difficulties people experience after injury to the brain and how sleep may be restorative. The glymphatic system, a cellular-waste removal system of lymphatic vessels attached to blood vessels, clears toxins from the central nervous system, including the amyloid beta protein (Aβ) implicated in Alzheimer's disease and the tau protein implicated in chronic traumatic encephalopathy (CTE) (see Chapter 4). The bottom line is that sleep may both restore function and prevent illness for everyone, perhaps especially for people with concussions or more severe TBIs.

In fact, sleep disturbances are much more common among people with TBI than for others. People with concussions may have had a preexisting problem sleeping. Overall functioning while awake can be severely affected after a concussion because sleep deprivation can exacerbate pain, memory problems, and mood disturbances. Some people experience events during sleep such as nightmares, especially if they have anxiety, post-traumatic stress disorder (PTSD), or panic disorder. Medications used before or after the concussion, including over-the-counter medications, can contribute to sleep problems. Lifestyle factors such as alcohol use, lack of physical activity, too-intense physical activity close to the time of sleep, or various stressors can contribute to sleep disturbances.

Concussions can cause a person to have difficulty falling asleep or staying asleep. Sometimes excessive daytime sleepiness occurs, and people with concussions may go on to have chronic insomnia, defined as insomnia that lasts more than three months. Circadian rhythm sleep-wake disorders and obstructive sleep apnea can also occur as a consequence of a TBI. Circadian rhythms are our bodies' twenty-four-hour clock cycles that influence physical and mental processes and behaviors, and that operate at the cellular level. The environment, especially light and darkness, and other cyclic behaviors such as eating or exercising influence these rhythms.

Genetic factors or factors that may affect body characteristics (such as a large neck circumference, excessive weight, an overbite, or a narrow airway) may also cause sleep difficulties. Cardiovascular disease, hypertension, diabetes mellitus, alcoholism, and smoking may predispose people to obstructive sleep apnea or another sleep disorder. Physicians must collect data about preexisting conditions like these, especially in older patients who have had concussions. For example, a driver may have nodded off and crashed into a tree because of an undiagnosed sleep disorder such as sleep apnea.

Managing Sleep Disturbances

Some activities can promote a good sleeping pattern, and the term "sleep hygiene" refers to these activities. Good sleep hygiene is more difficult than it seems. Many of us habitually underestimate the necessity of sleep. Exercising during the morning or afternoon, but not the evening, promotes sleep, and avoiding caffeine, alcohol, narcotics, and recreational drugs can also promote sleep and recovery after a concussion. Maintaining regular sleep-wake and meal times—called sleep stability—can also help; going to bed at the same time and getting up at the same time every day is essential to regularize sleep patterns and prevent insomnia. Tossing and turning for longer than fifteen to twenty minutes means it is time to stop trying and instead do something relaxing, such as reading or listening to relaxation tapes.

The bed should be used only for sleep and intimacy, and the bedroom should be safe, dark, quiet, and comfortable—this is called stimulus control. Whereas exposure to natural sunlight or shortwave (blue) light during the day can help to promote a good sleep pattern, these forms of light are not conducive to sleep at night. Electronic devices and LEDs emit blue light, types of artificial light that inhibit the secretion of the body's natural melatonin and the delta waves that promote sleep. Turning devices to a warm light mode in the evening may promote sleep. Amber glasses may help in the evening or early nighttime, as may sleep masks and earplugs if there are disturbing environmental conditions that cannot be altered.

Cognitive-behavioral therapy (CBT) uses a range of strategies to promote sleep stability. CBT includes a series of sleep assessments and advice about sleeping patterns and behaviors. A sleep diary can document patterns such as difficulty falling asleep or staying asleep, daytime drowsiness or napping, and factors that may contribute to disrupted sleep. The diary should reflect associated problems such as snoring, choking, gasping, or difficulty breathing, and abnormal movements or behaviors that a sleep partner might note and that might suggest sleep apnea or another medical problem. Morning headaches, memory difficulties, and mood changes can be linked to sleep apnea. In some cases, hormonal abnormalities—reduced thyroid hormone, testosterone, or growth hormone—or other factors might contribute to sleep problems and fatigue. Referral to a sleep medicine specialist is best for patients with chronic insomnia, circadian rhythm sleep-wake disorders, and obstructive sleep apnea. Smart phone apps can collect data, and sleep labs often send patients home with actigraph units.

Sleep apnea treatment usually requires airway pressure therapies with a continuous positive airway pressure (CPAP) machine. This effectively keeps the airway open with a flow of air. Surgery may be advised in some cases if there is an anatomic cause, such as the tongue or tissue in the back of the throat blocking the airway. Custom oral appliances can also be used to treat sleep apnea, and some people may tolerate these better than a CPAP machine.

Naps may help after a concussion, if they do not interfere with nighttime sleep. A short-term course of a sleep medication may be necessary in the early period, but drugs such as the benzodiazepines that affect memory should be avoided. Melatonin and ramelteon, a medication similar to melatonin, can treat insomnia, but should not be used for longer than thirty days. A physician should either prescribe or confirm the safety of any medication taken for sleep problems. For example, melatonin and ramelteon can interfere with other medications, such as antidepressants.

Shift work is notorious for disrupting workers' sleep-wake cycles, especially if the shifts are irregular or do not match a person's preferred sleep pattern. Nurses, physicians, and other health-care workers, police and firefighters, first responders, and truckers—all have an increased risk for sleep deprivation. Drowsy drivers can be perilous on the road, and people with concussions who are sleep-deprived are at risk to fall asleep at the wheel. Any work outside the interval of 7 a.m. to 6 p.m. is linked to poorer sleep, circadian-sleep disturbances, and additional stress in daily life.

The CDC's National Institute for Occupational Safety and Health (NIOSH) recommends regular rest of ten consecutive hours per day off-duty and rest breaks every one to two hours during demanding work. NIOSH recommends five eight-hour shifts, or four ten-hour shifts weekly; night shifts of no longer than eight hours are optimal. There should be one to two days off-schedule after each of these weekly shifts. For shift workers with concussions, schedules may need to change to facilitate recovery and to prevent another injury. Jason, the ER physician whose story began in Chapter 1, returned to work on an adjusted schedule, at first part-time, and then after three months, he returned to his usual twelve-hour shifts. By that time, his sleep cycles were regular again.

Managing Headaches

Every patient whose story appears in this book complained of headaches at some point during their treatment for concussion. That reminds us how common headaches are for people with concussions. In fact, most concussion patients report post-traumatic headaches (PTHs) that in some cases linger for months or even years. Oddly, people with more severe brain injuries experience fewer headaches than people with mild brain injuries or concussions. There is no clear evidence to explain this lower incidence. A PTH can begin immediately after a concussion or, more typically, within the first week. Any severe headache after a concussion that worsens or is accompanied by recurrent vomiting or a decreased level of awareness is a red flag that calls for an emergency evaluation. An orthostatic headache—one that worsens when standing—may also indicate a more serious problem that requires urgent care.

Subtypes of PTH include cervicogenic, migraine, and tension headaches. Injuries to peripheral nerves—occipital (back of the head) and supraorbital (top of the eye socket / eyebrow)—can also result in headaches. Cervicogenic and occipital neuralgia headaches are associated with neck pain, but a patient may experience the headache in the forehead. Patients often describe tension headaches as band-like pressure around the head and as mild to moderate in intensity. People who have migraine or migraine-like headaches can also have nausea, vomiting, sensitivity to light and sound, dizziness, insomnia, and even cognitive problems. Patients typically describe migraine headaches as throbbing.

If a patient had headaches before the concussion, they can worsen in intensity or frequency. Migraine headaches occur in 15 percent of adults, so some patients with concussions will have migraine history. In the general population, 75 percent of migraine sufferers are female. Scientists speculate that there may be a common biological mechanism between migraine and concussion. People who have fifteen or more days of headache during a month, with eight or more of those days including a migraine, have chronic migraine. People with fewer than fifteen days of headache in a month have episodic migraine.

Some studies suggest that those who serve in the armed forces who experience concussion from a blast or blunt injury have an even higher rate of migraine-type headaches than civilians who have a concussion. Jamie, an army lieutenant who suffered an injury in combat, had migraine headaches after the blast. He experienced flashing lights and often nausea. Migraine headaches are associated with a phenomenon called cortical spreading depression (a wave of cellular depolarization, or change in electrical charge, in the brain). (See Chapter 9 for more about Jamie's story.)

There are controversies about the prevalence of migraine headaches among people with PTH. Virginia physiatrist and brain injury medicine specialist Nathan Zasler offered his perspective to me on the diagnosis of PTH: "In my experience over more than three decades of practice, most headaches following concussion are not due to the concussion but rather to some combination of cervicogenic, musculoskeletal, and peripheral nerve injury. Other factors, including mood and sleep disorders (including depression, anxiety, and PTSD), stress, and medication overuse, may contribute. These headaches are often mixed and contributed to by more than one pain generator. A detailed headache history and complete physical exam of the face, head, neck and upper shoulders is critical prior to deciding on appropriate treatment. I won't tell you how many patients I see who have seen multiple physicians for their PTH and no one ever examined them above the shoulders."

Dr. Zasler believes that only about 20 percent of PTHs can be categorized as migraines. Most are cervicogenic. Soft tissue injuries such as whiplash, due to stretching of ligaments, or injury to other structures in the neck, such as a herniated cervical disc, can cause neck pain and related headaches. The injury to these structures can cause pain referred to the head, meaning the pain generator resides elsewhere but is felt in the head. Women have a higher incidence of cervicogenic headaches than men, perhaps because they also experience a higher frequency of whiplash.

With occipital neuralgia, the occipital nerve at the back of the head becomes stretched and irritated, causing pain and headaches, and a steroid injection can help. Pablo, the construction worker who fell from scaffolding, suffered severe headaches caused by occipital neuralgia and cervical strain (whiplash), and forehead pain above his right eye from injury to the supraorbital nerve. He had relief from injections of steroids for both problems. (See Chapter 9 for more of Pablo's story.) Some headaches, such as vestibular headaches, are triggered by eye or body movement. Evaluation by a neuro-ophthalmologist or neuro-optometrist experienced in treating people with brain injuries may be warranted if reading causes headaches, especially if they are associated with blurred vision.

A healthy diet, sleep, exercise, and stress management can help people with all headache types. Additional treatments combine biofeedback, stress management, relaxation training, cognitive-behavioral treatments, and trigger avoidance. A combination of treatment and self-management improves most headaches. Physical therapists can help treat cervicogenic PTHs. Tension headaches and even migraine headaches sometimes respond well to the older antidepressants such as amitriptyline or nortriptyline, or even over-the-counter acetaminophen. Nonsteroidal anti-inflammatories such as ibuprofen can be helpful with headaches, especially those caused by muscle or soft-tissue injuries of the neck, but dosing should be intermittent due to their potentially serious side effects, especially in older people. People who have had a concussion should avoid opioid medications for PTHs. Given the tragedy of the opioid epidemic, this advice merits repeating. Opioid medications can cause sedation, dizziness, vomiting, respiratory depression, and hormonal disorders such as low testosterone in addition to physical dependence and lethal consequences.

Physicians prescribe oral or intranasal triptans (serotonin stimulators) as a preventive approach at the very onset of a migraine headache. Triptans may take up to a month to become effective in this way. Propranolol (a beta-blocker that slows the heart rate) can sometimes be effective for preventing migraines. Patients with migraine headaches may have symptom relief from other medications such as gabapentin, topiramate, and valproate (drugs in the anticonvulsant or antiseizure class). Topiramate can be very effective, but it can also cause cognitive impairment, so this medication should be used with caution and under close observation. Injections with botulinum toxin (the neurotoxin produced by bacteria that cause botulism) may reduce the number of migraine attacks in some people.

Medication overuse headaches occur if a patient takes certain headache medications frequently (three or more times per week or more than fifteen days during a month) and for an extended period of time. They typically occur daily and on awakening, as medication effects wear off. Sometimes these rebound-type headaches come with cognitive problems or nausea. Treatment involves slowly withdrawing the medication, and the withdrawal can temporarily cause more severe headaches. Reducing the amount and frequency of medication and avoiding caffeine, a contributor to headaches in some people, can prevent these headaches.

Treatments vary considerably for the various types of posttraumatic headaches, so it is critical to diagnose the headache type. ER physician Jason's headaches were relieved with a low-dose antidepressant (amitriptyline) that also helped his sleep pattern. Pablo got relief from a combination of several nerve blocks (steroid injections at the back of his head and above his eye), gabapentin, and physical therapy. He still had tension headaches occasionally, but the shooting pains and nerve-related head and forehead pain resolved over a two-month period of treatment. Jamie, a veteran, received relief from the pain of migraine-type PTHs with acupuncture and manual therapy, relaxation exercises, and prophylactic treatment with a triptan prescribed by his VA neurologist. After ten months, his headaches became less frequent and less intense. Carla's headaches improved with prism glasses, along with vision exercises she performed at home, prescribed by her neuro-optometrist.

A PTH is considered chronic at three months. The medical literature suggests that up to one-third of patients still have headaches a year after a concussion. Given the fact that thorough physical examinations can go by the wayside, misdiagnosis may be a large part of the problem.

Managing Cognitive Symptoms

A person with a concussion may need to limit, though not necessarily eliminate, cognitive activities, including reading, writing, and working or going to school, at least in the early stages after injury. Activities that demand little attention may be gradually reintroduced for short periods of time, followed by gradual increases of both the demands of the activity and its duration. The inherent difficulty of a task, the concentration and speed required to complete it, the degree of familiarity with the task, and other factors dictate cognitive demand. For example, it is easier to read a magazine than to study for a calculus exam. Reading a text message is undemanding, but composing and sending multiple emails that require concentration in a stimulating environment might be very demanding. Action video games are highly cognitively demanding because of the response speed they call for. However, doing a jigsaw puzzle on a cell phone might be low demand.

Cognitive rehabilitation after a concussion treats people having problems with various brain functions that we depend on every day. This treatment focuses on the mental abilities that concussion most often affects—attention, concentration, and memory. But it might also take into account problems with executive function—comprehension, reasoning ability, problem solving, judgment, initiation, planning, and goal-setting. Cognitive rehabilitation interventions use exercises to restore function or strategies to help a person to compensate for mental difficulties. Treatment may emphasize techniques for solving problems in daily life through education and strategies for decision-making and accomplishing tasks.

Jason got help from his speech-language pathologist to learn cognitive strategies for organizing his work in the ER. She helped him realize that he had to take more notes when interviewing patients, and he needed a quiet space outside the chaotic ER venue to enter information and orders into the electronic medical record. Jason's neuropsychologist advised that he try a program of relaxation and mindfulness techniques for the anxiety that emerged when he had cognitive challenges. Over time, thanks to these education and treatment strategies, Jason returned to full-time work, and he earned a well-deserved promotion a year later.

Carla experienced many of the problems typical of young people who have had multiple concussions. She was easily overstimulated by her environment. The school hallway's fluorescent lights bothered her, so she wore a hat. She tried to avoid noisy, hectic locations like the cafeteria. Her attention problems made it difficult for her to focus on what she was reading or hearing. Little distractions caught her off guard, and she often lost her train of thought. She had trouble processing what happened in class, especially when the conversation went back and forth among many students, or when the teacher spoke quickly. Even working in small groups proved difficult for Carla. It helped to sit in the first row, but her classes involved a lot of memory work, and she had trouble recalling details to complete homework assignments and tests. Calculus was particularly difficult for Carla because of the complexity of the material and the multiple steps required to complete problems. English and history classes challenged her because she had trouble organizing her thoughts.

Carla's physician sent a letter to the school administration requesting additional accommodations—a 50 percent reduction in homework load, extra time for testing, deferral of standardized testing until the end of the school year when she had recovered, and a notetaker for her classes. The school assigned a classmate to take notes for her, although Carla tried her best to take down the main points of presentations and discussions. Carla's physician knew that Section 504 of the Rehabilitation Act of 1973 requires schools to conduct an assessment and requested one in a letter to the school. The school completed the 504 Plan with Carla and her parents. Carla also benefited from cognitive rehabilitation with a speech-language pathologist at the rehabilitation outpatient center. She learned compensation strategies, such as reorganizing her notes and her classmate's notes after class to reinforce her learning, and she used cognitive exercises, such as reading a paragraph and then writing down its details.

Medications that enhance certain mental functions, such as methylphenidate, a stimulant used primarily to treat attention deficit disorder / attention deficit hyperactivity disorder (ADD / ADHD), may help a limited number of people with cognitive problems after a concussion. Physicians usually prescribe these drugs in the chronic phases of treatment because recovery of mental functions can occur relatively quickly after a concussion, and medications always carry the risk of side effects. Sarah, whose childhood concussion was followed by a diagnosis of ADHD, found that going back on methylphenidate (a long-acting form), which she had not taken for years, helped her to focus and eventually return to work several months after the car crash.

Managing Sensory and Motor Symptoms

We sense information from our surroundings every millisecond of our conscious lives. Much of this sensing results in a motor response, termed a sensory-motor function. When we watch a basketball game, for example, our eyes move in relation to what is happening on the court, while the players use their highly developed sensory-motor abilities to play at high intensity. A sudden noise may make us turn to where our brain tells us the sound is coming from. Consider that when your bicycle hits a pothole and skids, you grip the handlebars, brace yourself, and hold steady. In one day of our lives, there are thousands of moments when we rely on our nervous system's sensory-motor functions, especially if we are performing skilled activities. But even seemingly simple activities such as walking or reading require intact sensory-motor pathways.

We take for granted that the sensory input from touch and our eyes and ears will not be confusing or debilitating; that is, until post-concussion symptoms emerge due to dysfunction of the vestibular-visual systems of the brain (see Chapter 1, Figure 6). Vestibular-visual symptoms include dizziness, vertigo, balance problems, and difficulty with visual fixation, focus, and tracking. Dizziness, balance problems, and headaches, which can be related to vestibular dysfunction, often accompany prolonged recoveries. Visual problems, such as blurred vision or double vision, occur in about a third of athletes who experience a concussion. Vestibulo-ocular reflex (VOR) gain, the change in the eye angle divided by the change in the head angle during a head turn, may be reduced after concussion, producing blurred vision.

Benign paroxysmal positional vertigo (BPPV), caused by dislodging tiny crystals in the inner ear, can also occur after a blow to the head or other forces that can cause a concussion. The crystals, called otoliths, in the utricle and saccule of the labyrinth (structures of the inner ear) live in a gel that has hair-like sensors for detecting linear movements (up and down and side to side) and relationship to gravity. When these crystals become dislodged into the adjacent semicircular canals (three looped structures that contain fluid and hair sensors that monitor the head's rotation), dizziness and vertigo occur, especially with movement. Physicians and physical therapists use a series of movements known as the Dix-Hallpike maneuver to diagnose BPPV, and the Epley maneuver to treat it.

Concussion may also cause a conductive hearing loss due to trauma to the tympanic membrane or the small bones in the middle ear—the incus, stapes, and anvil. These small bones, only a few millimeters in size, help transmit sound and language. Tinnitus (ringing or buzzing in the ears) also commonly occurs after concussion and may be related to shaking of the structures in the inner ear or to the brain. Change in the sense of smell can also occur with concussion, because the olfactory nerves are very exposed and vulnerable to injury, as are the olfactory centers in the brain itself. Anosmia (a lack of ability to smell odors) or dysosmia (a distortion of odors) affects a person's quality of life more than one might think, because in the absence of a sense of smell, food lacks flavor or can even become distasteful. It turns out that much of our appreciation of food is due to these olfactory systems, not our taste buds.

Judy, my patient who was thrown from her horse, lived with a number of debilitating problems after her concussion, including dizziness, tinnitus, a fear of losing her balance, photophobia (light sensitivity), an inability to smell cooking aromas, and blurry vision. She was dizzy traveling in a car, turning quickly, and bending over. She had trouble walking a straight line. Meclizine, a medication for dizziness, helped Judy's symptoms somewhat. Her gait slowed when she turned or tried to walk backward. She used a cane just to steady herself, and she always reached for handrails on stairs.

Judy's physical therapist found nystagmus (shaking of the eye during movements) using the Dix–Hallpike maneuver, suggesting BPPV. The therapist taught her the Epley maneuver to move the crystals back to their proper place. The therapist also taught her gaze and balance exercises she could do at home. Over a six-month period, Judy's balance and dizziness gradually improved, and she could walk steadily without a cane. An audiologist found Judy's hearing to be normal, and gradually her tinnitus went away with counseling, education, and cognitive behavioral therapy.

A neuro–optometrist found that Judy had problems with convergence and accommodation (focusing the eyes on a near object), eye gaze stabilization (fixating on an object), saccadic (quick) eye movements, and visual pursuit (smooth eye tracking), all of which interfered with her everyday life. Reading and looking at computer screens were difficult for Judy. These activities involve both eye tracking movements and saccades when her eyes moved from the end of one line to the beginning of the next or looked quickly from one part of the computer screen to another. Judy attended a few therapy sessions and received a program of home exercises that the neuro–optometrist called post-traumatic vision therapy. With this therapy, and by decreasing the brightness of her computer screen and increasing the font size, her blurred vision and difficulty focusing resolved. After twelve months, Judy was cleared to drive again. All of Judy's symptoms had resolved except for her sense of smell, which only partially returned.

Managing Emotional and Behavioral Symptoms

People commonly experience irritability after a concussion. Sometimes described in lay language as having a "short fuse," irritability can cause problems in relationships, especially for family members. It is important for those living with or those providing emotional support to people with post-concussion symptoms to be educated about this and offered strategies to help. More severe emotional problems such as anxiety, depression, and PTSD may occur. Rarely, patients may become suicidal. These conditions overlap with one another. Anxiety involves worry and fear, and sometimes panic, that might be generalized or specific to circumstances. Depression creates feelings of sadness, tearfulness, emptiness, or hopelessness, and loss of interest or pleasure in most or all normal activities.

PTSD symptoms may include recurrent nightmares or flashbacks about the incident, withdrawal or isolation, feelings of sadness or hopelessness, frequent thoughts about death or dying, or even serious thoughts about harm directed at self or others. Substance use (drug or alcohol) disorder can also prolong recovery and requires targeted treatments. Ongoing legal or insurance issues related to the concussion can cause stress or otherwise affect recovery. A concussion treatment plan should include evaluation and recommendations by a neuropsychologist if symptoms persist beyond a month, or earlier if symptoms suggesting PTSD, depression, or anxiety emerge. (See Chapters 2 and 9 for more discussions about PTSD.)

Persistent concussion symptoms often represent a complex interaction of psychological and physical factors, and it may not be possible to clearly distinguish among these. The uncertainty of having multiple symptoms without a clear explanation can lead even the most logical person to a cycle of frustration and preoccupation with their health. In fact, psychological problems such as anxiety and depression can make other symptoms worse, and effectively treating these conditions can lead to excellent outcomes. Often this entails more than one provider and good coordination of care. Individual psychotherapy using various approaches, group therapy, or support groups can help. Children often require psychoeducational interventions. Social workers can provide people with concussion and their families with techniques to improve family functioning or information about public or private resources, including support groups.

Jamie suffered a blast injury while serving in Afghanistan and received diagnoses of PTSD and chronic pain. His mental health treatment involved intensive psychotherapy, eye-movement desensitization and reprocessing (EMDR), assignment of a mental health service animal, and an antidepressant. He also received a diagnosis of an endocrine disorder from the blast injury—low growth hormone and low testosterone. He was prescribed hormone replacement therapy that improved his mood, ability to focus, level of fatigue, and sexual functioning. His service animal, Toby, made him feel safe and supported, and relaxation techniques, mindfulness, and art therapy helped his recovery.

Sarah's history of anxiety worsened after the concussion she experienced during a car crash. Cognitive-behavioral therapy and buspirone (a medication for anxiety) helped her. A program of aerobic exercise at a local gym improved her mood and her thinking skills. Her recovery was prolonged, but nine months after the car crash, she was able to work again.

Final Thoughts

As with any medical condition, correct diagnosis is the only path to effective treatment. The good news is that options exist for people with concussion and post-concussion symptoms to help them recover, using a variety of no-harm or least-harm treatments. Finding a treatment setting with an interdisciplinary approach, such as a rehabilitation center or comprehensive concussion clinic staffed with skilled and knowledgeable physicians and other health-care providers is the best route for people whose symptoms do not resolve relatively quickly.

Some recovery of brain functions that have been injured in a concussion happens naturally through neuroplasticity, or adaptation. We do not yet understand these processes well enough to improve these functions through specific interventions, although there is evidence that exercise and sleep may help. Nutrition and dietary supplements may also be helpful alternative treatments, but we do not have sufficient evidence to recommend these or any of the raft of new technological interventions that manufacturers and investigators are marketing.

For those who have suffered multiple concussions, prognosis must be guarded. Outcomes depend on many factors: the severity and recovery times for each concussion, age at the time of injury, and genetics. Chapter 4 presents troubling data to suggest that some in this group with recurrent concussions, including a substantial number of athletes of all ages, will live with long-term consequences.

4

Long-Term Risks

I n 1869, Princeton and Rutgers played in the first American college football game, introducing the new sport as a hybrid of soccer and rugby. Seventeen years later, in 1876, Yale rugby player Walter Camp wrote the first set of football rules, and college football pushed the sport to dominance, paving the way for the first professional team to form in 1897. The *New York Times* minced no words in the paper's 1893 story about this new American sport: "Change the Football Rules: The Rugby Game as Played Now Is a Dangerous Pastime." Historian Emily Harrison chronicles this and other news articles that made the case for football's extreme risks. She documents how the sport's promoters sidelined facts about player injuries, noting similarities to how the National Football League (NFL) delayed acknowledging its concussion problem in the twenty-first century (see Chapter 7).

Scientists and health-care providers have known about the dangers of repeat concussions, immediate and in the long term, especially for boxers and football players, for many decades. Medical historians also began decades ago to uncover a wealth of evidence about the inherent risks of these two sports. Boxing is unequivocally a combat sport, and football entails deliberate, violent collisions between players. In fact, we now call football a collision sport rather than simply a contact sport, acknowledging the game's inherent violence.

In 1906, two surgeons at Boston City Hospital, Edward Nichols and Homer Smith, reported the Harvard football team's high injury rates in the *Boston Medical and Surgical Journal*. In "The Physical Aspect of American Football," an article responding to the death of a Harvard football player that same year, Harrison notes that Nichols and Smith "highlighted one injury in particular that had been hiding in plain sight: concussion of the brain." In 1915, the editors of the *Journal of the American Medical Association (JAMA)* warned: "events which depend for thrill on the nearest possible approach to death by the actors in them represent the degeneracy which overtakes sport and makes madness of it." Charles W. Eliot, president of Harvard University, pressed for an end to college football in response to its dangers.

Although he spoke out about severe injuries and deaths suffered by college football players, President Theodore Roosevelt is credited with saving the game. An avid fan, he helped bring the Ivy League schools together to push for rule changes to make the game safer. Sports historian Allen Guttmann pointed out the cultural issues inherent in Roosevelt's advocacy: "Football had a long career as the chosen sport of Ivy League athletes eager to prove that they were real men and not the 'mollycoddles' ridiculed by Theodore

Roosevelt and other upper-class exponents of the 'strenuous life.'"
Roosevelt's advocacy did prompt the creation of the National Collegiate Athletic Association (NCAA) in 1906. Some of the key rule additions and changes to American football that followed included establishing a line of scrimmage, eliminating body-breaking mass formations, increasing the first-down distance from five to ten yards, and introducing the forward pass.

American football grew exponentially in popularity beginning in the final decades of the nineteenth century. The American Professional Football Association formed in 1920, becoming the NFL two years later. Deaths due to brain and spinal cord injuries continued to occur at high rates during the decades that followed. Nevertheless, by the 1960s, more and more boys and young men were playing the sport. In a much-publicized case, New York Giants running back Frank Gifford suffered a major brain injury in 1960 that eventually ended his twelve-year football career in 1964. Gifford's prominent retirement was not enough to produce major changes in how the game was played. Football had begun its reign as America's favorite sport, and Gifford switched careers to actor and sports commentator. Gifford died at the age of 84 in 2015. Later that year, his family disclosed his postmortem diagnosis: chronic traumatic encephalopathy (CTE).

Punch Drunk and Other Labels

While football dominates the concussion news today, boxing was the first sport to raise brain health concerns for its athletes, concerns that surfaced during the nineteenth century. Descended from gladiatorial spectacles, this ancient sport gained legitimacy in 1867 when England adopted the Marquess of Queensberry rules that, despite opposition on both sides of the Atlantic, paved the way for the modern boxing era in Europe and the United States. Boxers target the head, and loss of consciousness is the sport's primary objective. Hence, it was easier to make the case for a link between this sport and neurodegenerative diseases (NDs) in one-on-one combat than for the team sport of football.

In 1928, New Jersey physician and medical examiner Harrison Martland noted that fans talked about boxers having a condition they dubbed "punch drunk"—acting inebriated from being hit in the head rather than from drinking. Martland examined twenty-three former boxers and recorded gait unsteadiness, physical slowness, tremors, and speech problems. He observed that "the occurrence of the symptoms in almost 50 per cent of fighters who develop this condition in mild or severe form, if they keep at the game long enough, seems to be good evidence that some special brain injury due to their occupation exists." All but one of these fighters also experienced cognitive problems— mental slowing and periods of confusion. Although Martland de- scribed many of these cases as mild and not progressive, he observed that "in severe cases, there may develop a peculiar tilting of the head, a marked dragging of one or both legs, a staggering, propulsive gait with the facial characteristics of the parkinsonian syndrome, or a backward swaying of the body, tremors, vertigo and deafness." He added a chilling statement: "Finally, marked mental deterioration may set in necessitating commitment to an asylum."

As more physicians observed progressive neurologic and behav- ioral impairments in boxers, they coined new terms to describe these conditions. In 1927, psychiatrists Michael Osnato and Vincent Giliberti published a study of 100 boxers with progressive neuro- logical diseases. They found headaches, dizziness, and neurologic signs, and they named this condition "traumatic encephalitis." Os- nato and his colleague H. L. Parker used the term "traumatic en- cephalopathy," and US Navy physician J. A. Millspaugh coined the term "dementia pugilistica" in the late 1930s.

In 1940, psychiatrists Karl Murdoch Bowman and Abram Blau described a twenty-eight-year-old professional boxer who had poor insight, paranoia, and memory difficulties. Their chapter in Brock's 1940 textbook *Injuries of the Skull, Brain and Spinal Cord,* called "Psychotic States Following Head and Brain Injury in Adults and Children," outlined a system for classifying mental disorders caused by traumatic brain injury (TBI). Bowman and Blau named the boxer's disorder chronic traumatic encephalopathy (CTE). In due time, CTE would be the name that stuck to designate the unique, long-term effects of repeat concussions in football players and other athletes.

In 1949, the world-renowned neurologist MacDonald Critchley described similar findings in a boxer in his mid-50s. Critchley published an extensive study of sixty-nine boxers in 1957, describing behavior remarkably similar to that of high-profile former football players in twenty-first-century news media. The boxers Critchley examined had memory and speech problems and sometimes dementia, poor insight, depression, emotional lability, paranoia, disinhibition, and aggression. They also suffered from intractable headaches, dizziness, and an unsteady gaze. Critchley found neurofibrillary (NF) tangles (abnormal proteins) in those boxers' brains. He described this condition as CTE.

The neurologist who coined the term "accident neurosis" for post-concussion symptoms, Henry Miller, weighed in about CTE in a publication of the Royal Society of Medicine in 1966. He noted that repetitive brain injuries lead to widespread atrophy (loss of brain tissue), especially in the frontal lobes; cellular changes characteristic of Alzheimer's disease; and a rare finding of a midline cavity in the brain—a communicating dilated cavum septum pellucidum (a membrane between the corpus callosum and the fornix that has been called "the fifth ventricle"). The dilated cavum septum can occur as a congenital anomaly when the membrane fails to close fully during fetal development, but it also is found in some boxers' brains.

Pathologist Anthony Herber Roberts studied a random sample of more than 200 retired boxers professionally registered in England between 1929 and 1955. These fighters had extensive exposure to neurotrauma from participating in hundreds of professional bouts during boxing careers lasting up to twenty years. Many had CTE, a disorder Roberts described as affecting movement and also causing confusion, memory loss, dementia, and aggressive behaviors. Roberts calculated that about one in ten boxers has at least a mild form of CTE, and one in twenty a moderate-to-severe form of the disorder.

In 1906, around the time that football surged in popularity in the United States, psychiatrist and neuropathologist Alois Alzheimer reported autopsy findings from the brain of a 55-year-old German woman, Auguste Deter. She died with a progressive cognitive and behavioral disorder, and Alzheimer found NF tangles and amyloid plaques (abnormal clusters of protein) in her brain, the hallmarks of the disease that now bears his name.

In 1990, using updated techniques, British neuropathologist Gareth Roberts re-examined the brains of boxers with dementia pugilistica, the same brains that another British neuropathologist, John Corsellis, had studied in the 1970s. Corsellis had discovered NF tangles in these brains, but Roberts found that almost all these boxers' brains contained additional plaques typical of Alzheimer's disease. Roberts concluded that it was probable that this disease and dementia pugilistica share common pathological mechanisms. By the twenty-first century, this story was poised to migrate onto the football field.

Gareth Roberts and his colleagues also conducted a pathological study of the brain of "a punch-drunk wife" and published their results in the *Lancet* in 1990. This obscure case report tells the tale of what may happen with repetitive concussions or more serious TBIs from domestic violence (now referred to as intimate partner violence): CTE (see Chapter 8).

Football No Longer Sidelined

Heavyweight champion Muhammad Ali moved stiffly and with a visible tremor as he lit the torch at the 1996 Olympic Games in Atlanta, Georgia, a television image that remains indelible in many minds. Born Cassius Clay, Ali grew up in the Jim Crow–segregated South. He entered the boxing world as a teenager, making the US team in 1960 for the Olympic Games in Rome. Some neurologists still debate whether Ali's parkinsonism resulted from repetitive concussions or from genetics, but the torch lighting made public the link between brain injuries and NDs.

The culture surrounding America's favorite sport of football balked at this link, however. Football fans had grown accustomed to watching "dinged" players stagger off the field, but they weren't yet willing to connect the damage associated with hits in boxing, a combat sport, to football, merely a collision sport. While a few football players with evidence of neurologic decline appeared in medical or scientific journals in the 1930s, it would be seventy years before the public, and for that matter the medical community, fully acknowledged football's link to CTE and other NDs.

In 2005, Pittsburgh pathologist Bennet Omalu reported what he described as a sentinel case of CTE in a football player. After Pittsburgh Steelers center Mike Webster's death in 2002 at the age of 50, Omalu's postmortem examination revealed signs of an extensive ND. Omalu found widespread accumulations of an abnormal protein called phosphorylated tau (p-tau), tau with the addition of a phosphate group. P-tau was the same abnormal protein found in boxers' brains. Omalu's findings suggested that a devastating brain disorder explained the severe cognitive and behavioral problems that derailed Webster's life.

Omalu and his colleague Steven DeKosky, an Alzheimer's disease expert, used the methods of neuropathologist James Geddes to verify tauopathy, the hallmark signs of dementia pugilistica. Understandably, they deemed dementia pugilistica an inaccurate name for a disease that did not affect only boxers. As DeKosky told *MedPage Today:* "We didn't want to call it dementia pugilistica because Webster wasn't a boxer. We spent a lot of time thinking about it and came up with chronic traumatic encephalopathy (CTE) as the name, because dementia footballistica doesn't have a ring to it. That terminology was used in the 70s to describe it, but it had been lost." As we learned, the term CTE was actually coined in the 1940s, and neurologic disorders associated with boxing were identified even decades prior to that.

Omalu submitted his paper to the journal *Neurosurgery,* and the journal's reviewer, rheumatologist Elliot Pellman, who was also the chair of the NFL's Mild Traumatic Brain Injury Committee, initially rejected it. Pellman and the journal later agreed to publish the 2005 report, but they also published a letter to the editor written by Pellman, Ira Casson, and David Viano, all members of the NFL committee. DeKosky called the letter "a hostile, insulting commentary." Supportive letters poured in from prominent leaders in neurosurgery and neuropsychology in response, and Omalu and his colleagues kept up their scientific pursuit of CTE. In 2006, *Neurosurgery* published another CTE case, that of Steelers' lineman Terry Long, who had committed suicide at age 45.

The public began to learn a lot about football, concussions, and CTE as journalists picked up these case reports, noted the NFL resistance to their importance, and ramped up their reporting.

High-profile news articles, books, and movies brought into clear focus the interconnections between money, politics, sports, and medicine (see Chapter 7). From 2006 to 2011, the prolific *New York Times* journalist Alan Schwarz produced a steady stream of more than a hundred articles about concussions, the NFL, and the dangers of football.

Schwarz's first story concerned Philadelphia Eagles' safety Andre Waters, who committed suicide in 2007 at the age of 44, and in whose brain Omalu found extensive evidence of CTE. Schwarz is largely responsible for raising global awareness about the risks of football and other collision sports and with moving the NFL from denial to action. The NFL feared that revelations about CTE could kill the sport as well as create a potential liability nightmare. In 2007, the NFL finally enacted league-wide guidelines and rules regulating post-concussion medical treatment and return-to-play standards, and the media buzz probably had a lot to do with this development. The changes, sadly, came far too late for retired football players from the 1970s, 1980s, and 1990s, many of whom are not eligible for medical benefits according to these rules.

In 2013, ESPN reporters and brothers Mark Fainaru-Wada and Steve Fainaru published *League of Denial,* a bestseller that followed the release of a documentary of the same name shown on PBS's *Frontline.* The authors retrospectively explored the story of CTE and professional football, beginning in 1974 at the start of Mike Webster's career. The authors weaved in the stories of other NFL players, such as Dave Duerson and Junior Seau, who both committed suicide and were posthumously diagnosed with CTE. The reporters compared the NFL's role to that of tobacco companies that refused to acknowledge any relationship between lung cancer and cigarette

smoking, thus exposing the dark, profit-first side of America's favorite sport.

Journalist Jeanne Marie Laskas helped to make Bennet Omalu's
and Mike Webster's stories public, first with an article in *GQ* in
2009. Her 2015 book *Concussion* chronicles Omalu's life and struggles, from his childhood in Nigeria to his training and practice as a
forensic pathologist in the United States. In the 2015 film made from
the book, Will Smith plays Bennet Omalu. The film screened in
mainstream movie theaters across the United States. Like the book,
the film dramatizes the story of Mike Webster and the NFL's subsequent attempts to avoid what became known as the concussion
crisis.

Laskas also unearthed earlier NFL stories. Jets wide receiver Al
Toon and Steelers running back Merril Hoge both retired in the
1990s at age 29 after suffering many concussions on the field. On
one Sunday alone in 1994, three quarterbacks lost consciousness on
football fields. Laskas, also speaking for Omalu, hit this nail on the
head:

> The PR was terrible for America's game. Good clean fun.
> Family fun that began with pee wee leagues in towns and
> farms and suburbs of America. High school dreams and
> leather jackets and cheerleaders bouncing. And then the
> NFL! Not just a league but a whole entertainment industry.
> Bigger than any other sport. Way bigger. Bigger than TV.
> Bigger than music. Bigger than Hollywood. An 8 billion
> per year American success story. The hits were part of the
> fun. Fans loved them. The NFL sold "Greatest Hits" video-
> tapes at Kmart for people who wanted to watch them again
> and again.

Brain Banks

Omalu's first discovery of CTE in the dissected brain of Mike Webster propelled additional research and the establishment of brain banks to study CTE and other NDs. Ann McKee has now identified many CTE cases, beginning in 2009 with the publication of the first forty-eight cases. McKee is chief neuropathologist for the New England Veterans Administration Medical Centers (VAMCs) and also director of the Boston University brain banks at the Bedford, Massachusetts, VAMC. Brain banks such as these study a select group—those who have voluntarily marked their brains for donation, or whose next of kin make the donation because they suspect that the athletic career of their loved one caused neurologic problems. CTE is found in these brains at a higher rate than would affect a more random sample of former players.

In a large study of the brains of 202 former football players in 2017, Boston University neurologist and Alzheimer's researcher Jesse Mez, Ann McKee, and their colleagues found that 177, or nearly 88 percent, of these brains show evidence of CTE. Most are the brains of semiprofessional and professional players with a median age of 66 and fifteen years of football participation. Only one of the 111 NFL players' brains and only one of the eight Canadian Football League (CFL) players' brains lacked evidence of CTE. The researchers found severe pathology in nine of ten professional players and six of ten former college and semiprofessional players. Early-stage CTE was also found in three of fourteen high school football players.

Boston University biomedical engineer Chad Tagge, psychiatrist Lee Goldstein, and their collaborators further explored CTE in a study of four teenage athletes who suffered impacts to the head but were not clinically diagnosed with concussions. Their brains contained activated astrocytes, neuronal destruction, and tau accumulations around blood vessels. This led the team to explore CTE using an animal research model, and they discovered that even impacts not strong enough to cause overt concussion signs may lead to tauopathy.

Jorge Barrio, Bennet Omalu, and colleagues have used positron emission tomography (PET) imaging in an attempt to diagnose CTE in a living patient. This technique is still considered experimental. At this time, CTE can be diagnosed only after death through a brain autopsy and corresponding pathologic investigations.

Introducing Amyloid and Tau

As the story of CTE in boxers and football players continues to unfold, it is clear that CTE intersects with other NDs, especially Alzheimer's. Amyloid is a protein aggregate associated with many diseases affecting various organs and systems of the human body. Amyloid β (Aβ) is a form of this protein found in the brain and spinal cord. We do not yet fully understand its function, but it likely plays a role in both brain development and neuroplasticity. It is also a culprit in Alzheimer's disease. Amyloid diseases such as Alzheimer's are triggered in part by an inflammatory process, similar in a basic way to arthritis or a sore throat. A cellular event, perhaps due to genetics, the environment, or a combination of both, may activate the process of overproduction of amyloid precursor protein (APP). These substances accumulate in the brain's axons and synapses and overwhelm its cellular apparatus.

Damaged axons eventually expel Aβ, and it turns into plaques outside the cell, leading to the brain destruction that psychiatrist and neuropathologist Alois Alzheimer discovered. Neurons lose their ability to function and their synaptic connections with other neurons. Many neurons die, causing the brain to atrophy or shrink.

Amyloid β plaques sometimes occur in middle-aged and older adults who have mild cognitive deterioration, or even no cognitive or psychological problems, but not to the extent found in those with NDs.

Looking at brain tissue for CTE under a microscope reveals a different complex pathology, but with one constant—an abnormality related to another protein called tau. The nerve cell's apparatus—the microtubes, axonal transport systems, and cell-signaling pathways—requires tau protein for support. Brain injury can result in elevations of tau protein in the cerebrospinal fluid (CSF), making it a potential biomarker for CTE. Tau deposits characterize late Alzheimer's and frontotemporal dementia (formerly called Pick's disease). Tau also appears in normal aging, but not with the distinct pattern and distribution its pathology takes on in CTE.

Tau pathology or tauopathy proceeds in a stepwise progression. It likely begins with inflammation and the activation of kinase (an enzyme that catalyzes phosphorylation—the transfer of a phosphate group). This is known as the p-tau event. Then p-tau protein accumulates to form chemical complexes and produce NF tangles, ultimately resulting in massive destruction of brain tissue. Chronic inflammation, also fueling the disease, keeps the destruction going.

There is evidence that trauma can make tau go haywire and cause this protein to behave like the prions (misfolded proteins) described in Creutzfeldt-Jakob disease (mad cow disease in humans). Prions propagate themselves and have high latency, meaning that they work their destruction over time. These abnormal proteins start in one place and progressively move to other parts of the brain. The rogue form of tau—cis-tau—damages the microtubules and mitochondria and may link brain trauma to both Alzheimer's disease and CTE.

Harvard Medical School researcher Asami Kondo and his team discovered an antibody to cis-tau that might lead to preventing and treating NDs. Research on the link between acute TBI and CTE now intensely focuses on the endoplasmic reticulum, that protein-manufacturing center for the cell labeled with Nissl stain by early researchers (see Chapter 1 and Figure 1). West Virginia School of Medicine's Brandon Lucke-Wold and his collaborators are investigating this link in a search for treatments.

CTE Stages

In milder cases of CTE, the brain can appear almost normal to pathologists. In severe cases, the brain atrophies and its ventricles enlarge, which also occurs in Alzheimer's. The corpus callosum becomes thin, and the nearby septum pellucidum exhibits abnormalities just like those observed by early researchers in boxers' brains. The cerebellum shows scarring and evidence of neuronal loss. Abnormalities in CTE brains are localized to superficial cortical layers and in the depths of sulci (grooves on the brain surfaces), and the pathology is perivascular (around the blood vessels) and periventricular (around the ventricles that contain CSF). These are the areas of the brain most susceptible to the stress and strain caused by inertial forces. The characteristic tau locations might be predicted by scientists' observations of diffuse axonal injury (DAI), although DAI has its own stepwise cellular damage process (see Chapter 1 and Figure 2).

The National Institutes of Health held a consensus conference in 2016 to begin to standardize CTE pathology classification. Attendees agreed that Stage 1 CTE involves small focal perivascular epicenters of p-tau, tangles in epicenters at the depths of the sulci, and some axonal loss in the frontal and temporal lobes. The frontal lobes, the seat of our higher-level reasoning abilities required for decision-making, judgment, and problem-solving, are among the first areas to be affected. In Stage 1, an affected person may experience no clinical symptoms, or only minor symptoms such as headaches, difficulty concentrating, and mild mood changes.

Stage 1 affects the locus coeruleus (LC), a key structure in the brainstem that forms part of the reticular activating system (RAS), the system that keeps us awake and alert. This structure also serves as a major relay station, receiving input from the cingulate cortex and the amygdala. These structures are involved in pain, emotional regulation and behavior, and stress signaling. The LC connects with many other areas of the brain, including the frontal lobes and hippocampus, and damage to the LC can therefore impair cognitive processes involving attention, memory, and decision-making.

In Stage 2 brains, the tau pathology has spread to multiple parts of the frontal, temporal, and parietal lobes. The thalamus and hypothalamus, deeper within the brain, also show tauopathy. By Stage 2, people with CTE have more difficulty managing their emotions and show more problems with thinking and memory. They may have mood swings, depression, and problems with language, such as difficulty finding the right words.

The Stage 3 CTE brain shows widespread and dense tau pathology, again especially in the frontal and temporal lobes (see Figure 7). The nucleus basalis of Meynert, a region that has functions related to attention and memory, enriched with the neurotransmitter acetylcholine, is devastated with tauopathy by this stage. This region can also be affected in people with Alzheimer's disease, Parkinson's disease, and frontotemporal dementia. Some Stage 3 cases show cavum septum pellucidum (collapse of this membrane between the hemispheres), a finding in dementia pugilistica (boxer's CTE). In Stage 3 CTE, headaches, attention and concentration problems, memory loss, executive function impairments, dementia, mood and behavioral disorders, suicidality, language and visuo-perceptual impairments, and movement disorders are often prominent features.

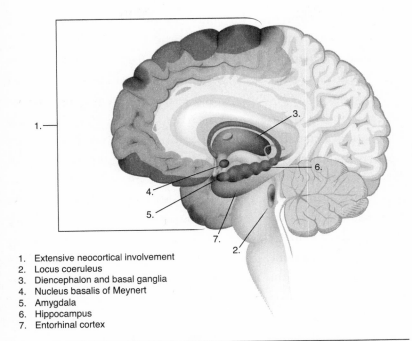

1. Extensive neocortical involvement
2. Locus coeruleus
3. Diencephalon and basal ganglia
4. Nucleus basalis of Meynert
5. Amygdala
6. Hippocampus
7. Entorhinal cortex

FIGURE 7 Stage 3 chronic traumatic encephalopathy (CTE) with widespread and dense tau pathology.

In Stage 4, people can experience severe dementia symptoms that can be similar to those stemming from Alzheimer's or Parkinson's disease. In this final stage, the pathology spreads to most regions of the cerebral cortex, the hippocampus, and the amygdala. Atrophy is more severe, with extensive DAI and gliosis (reaction of glial cells and scarring), and ventriculomegaly (enlargement of the ventricles, the chambers in the brain that hold and circulate cerebrospinal fluid). Ann McKee and her Boston University colleagues found that only slightly more than half of the subjects in this Stage 4 group show "pure" CTE. The remaining brains show additional neuropathological findings associated with Alzheimer's, or microscopic findings of much rarer NDs such as frontotemporal dementia, Lewy body dementia, or amyotrophic lateral sclerosis (ALS).

McKee's group, including neurologist Robert Stern, has collaborated with other research groups and the National Institutes of Health to refine CTE subtypes. These subtypes seem to fit with the clinical descriptions of boxers by early researchers. The first boxer subtype is young and has behavior and mood problems. The other type is an older boxer. These individuals are depressed, moody, apathetic, aggressive, and impulsive. They have memory and executive function impairments, and ultimately dementia. Movement problems such as stiffness and slowness, dysarthria (slurred speech), and ataxia (balance problems) occur in some with the advanced disease, similar to the symptoms of Parkinson's disease.

The differences and similarities among NDs, their relationship to each other and to genetics and the environment, present a puzzle that has yet to be solved. Questions remain about how these conditions overlap and how to classify them. Columbia University researcher Patricia Washington and her team ask a big question in their 2015 article: "Does brain injury trigger distinct NDs, or should they be classified together as traumatic encephalopathy?" Australian researcher Andrew Gardner and his colleagues reported that only one-fifth of eighty-five cases of athletes autopsied over a ten-year period had "pure" neuropathology consistent with CTE alone; about half had CTE plus other neuropathology, and about one-quarter had no neuropathology. Others have challenged these findings, and the debates continue.

Broadening the scope of the potential population of people with late effects of repetitive concussions under the category "Traumatic Encephalopathy Syndrome" (TES), as University of Michigan researcher Nicole Reams and her colleagues suggest, might go too far. Harvard neuropsychologist Grant Iverson and his colleagues assert:

"This syndrome is extraordinarily broad in scope, encompassing people with mild depression and those with late-stage dementia. For example, if a person played high school and collegiate sports (for at least two years at the college level) and had current problems with depression, anxiety, and headaches, that person would meet criteria for the new Traumatic Encephalopathy Syndrome."

Partly Our Genes

Scientists have long suspected that genetics may set the stage for progressive diseases of the brain. Alzheimer's, the most common cause of dementia in the world and therefore the most studied of the NDs, clearly has a genetic component. For reasons we do not yet understand, women make up almost two-thirds of those diagnosed with Alzheimer's, but aging represents the most important risk factor for the disease, with a doubling of risk every five years after age 65.

Every human cell contains DNA instructions packed into its chromosomes. Each chromosome holds many genes, the codes that define our individual human characteristics and provide direction for cell activities. Each human cell contains two copies of each chromosome, and DNA makes up both. An allele is an alternate form of a gene, and alleles on the two chromosomes might be the same (homozygous state) or different (heterozygous state). We can inherit genetic mutations from our parents, or they can occur after birth. Mutations can carry high risks for certain diseases. Early-onset Alzheimer's provides one example.

Genetic variants—differences in genes—may increase or decrease a person's risk of developing a disease or condition. We call these susceptibility genes or genetic risk factors. The gene for apolipoprotein (Apo) is a case in point. Apo makes up a main component of lipoproteins in blood plasma and functions in important ways to guide cholesterol and lipid transport. The liver and astrocytes in the brain synthesize Apo. Apo plays a primary role in lipid delivery for growing and regenerating axons after a neuronal injury.

The three major Apo alleles—E2, E3, and E4—differ in their effects. E2 and possibly E3 protect against Alzheimer's, while E4 represents a definite risk factor for the disease. An E4 / E4 pattern (homozygous state) carries more risk than E4 / E3 or E4 / E2 (two different heterozygous states). People with one copy of E4, about one in five of us, have up to five times the risk of developing the disease compared to people without the variant, and they develop the disease earlier. People with two copies, just 2 percent of the population, bear up to fifteen times the risk. About 90 percent of people with two copies of E4 will develop Alzheimer's by the time they reach the age of 80. Ten percent of early-onset cases of Alzheimer's, diagnosed between the ages of 30 and 60, are caused by different genetic mutations on different chromosomes than late-onset Alzheimer's. The ultimate effects—Aβ plaques and devastating cognitive and behavioral impairments—are the same.

An injury to the brain can trigger Aβ accumulations, just as aging can. Early studies establishing a link between TBI and Alzheimer's came from Glasgow researchers Gareth W. Roberts and his colleagues in the 1990s. They found that about 30 percent of people who die early from severe TBI, even children, have these plaques. The unhappy combination of a genetic heritage of an ApoE4 allele and a history of TBI may result in a staggering tenfold increased risk of developing Alzheimer's.

In the 1990s, New York neurologist Barry Jordan studied boxers' genetic susceptibilities to late-life brain disorders. He found that boxers who carry the ApoE4 allele are more likely to experience cognitive difficulties and to develop a chronic disorder that shares many characteristics with Alzheimer's. All of the severely impaired boxers he studied had at least one ApoE4 allele and had dysarthria and ataxia. Some of the boxers also had disinhibition, irritability, euphoria or hypomania, impaired insight, paranoia, and violent outbursts. Jordan identified a spectrum of cognitive problems ranging from mild disorders to dementia.

Jordan conjectured that these problems may result from personality traits, aging, an ND, or some combination of these factors, and that genetics probably plays a key role. A long boxing career, high exposure rates (number of bouts and sparring), and many knockouts, along with tolerating many blows without being knocked out, seems to increase the possibility of a dire outcome.

The presence of the ApoE4 allele may predispose people to more cognitive problems or greater numbers of symptoms after a concussion. This was a finding in a number of studies, including one of athletes led by Victoria Merritt and Peter Arnett at Penn State University. Genetics remains a rich area of study for understanding risks for athletes and others who undergo repetitive concussions.

Big Data Studies

Researchers who study the associations between NDs and TBI have worked with laboratory animals, used brain bank data, or collected and mined observational (nonexperimental) and retrospective (based on data already collected) data for analysis. Each of these research methods brings inherent strengths along with some weaknesses. Animal research methods vary widely, and findings in animals may not apply to humans. Convenience samples (subjects who happen to be available, such as clinic patients or volunteers) can provide evidence about selected groups, but such samples cannot ultimately support conclusions about incidence or risk. Brain banks also contain selective samples from what are called opportunistic cohorts, and bank researchers usually collect data from family members after the death of the person under study. Recall bias (an error caused by inaccurately remembering an event or experience) by a person being studied or a family member can skew results.

Very large databases may not contain the right data elements to answer important questions or make significant comparisons between populations. Researchers sometimes use different definitions or terms, or different measures of severity or outcome. Coding systems and populations often vary from one study to the next. Observational studies looking for risk examine what is called relative risk, usually between two populations. Sometimes these studies use a comparatively short period of measurement, and this weakens conclusions. And relative risk is not the same as absolute risk, which calculates a person's lifetime chance of developing a disease, because absolute risk is much smaller than relative risk. The possibility of reverse causation may throw results into question as well. For example, did the TBI cause the disease, or was something else the cause, such as a lifestyle factor, a genetic trait, or a not-yet-diagnosed disease? For all these reasons, researchers must be wary about drawing firm conclusions from observational studies, especially about what causes NDs. Looking at all the research into NDs, it's hard not to feel confused. Laboratory scientists, clinical researchers, and practicing physicians continue to debate these issues surrounding concussion and neurodegenerative diseases.

Dementia and TBI

Despite these shortcomings, population studies decades ago found individuals with a history of TBI incur a two to four times increased risk of developing Alzheimer's. In 1989, psychologist Angela Gedye and her University of British Columbia collaborators found that people who have a severe TBI before the age of 65 and who develop Alzheimer's experience symptom onset eight years earlier than

Alzheimer's patients with no history of a TBI. Ten years later, another study by British Columbia researcher Peter Nemetz showed TBI to be linked to an accelerated time to onset of Alzheimer's. During the 1990s, Boston University neurologist Z. Guo and the Multi-Institutional Research in Alzheimer's Genetic Epidemiology (MIRAGE) team also found an increased risk of Alzheimer's in patients with a history of TBI, with greater risk for those patients whose injuries were more severe, or who lost consciousness. They also found a greater risk among first-degree relatives (parents, siblings, or children) of Alzheimer's patients.

More recently, epidemiologists Anna and Peter Nördstrom used a large Swedish database of people over 50, segregating the data into three cohorts using controls and sibling pairs. Using both a retrospective and a case–control approach (comparing outcomes of people with dementia and people without), they found a four to five times increased risk of dementia in the first year after a TBI. The risk decreased in later years, but it remained significant for more than thirty years following the injury and was still higher than for controls in the mild TBI or concussion group. The sibling cohort, those brothers and sisters without a history of a TBI, strengthened these results.

University of California San Francisco (UCSF) neurologist and epidemiologist Raquel Gardner investigated dementia from any cause in a large database of US patients with TBI using a control population of patients exposed to trauma without a TBI. Those with a moderate to severe injury had an increased risk of dementia for up to seven years, and even a single, mild TBI increased the risk of dementia in patients who were sixty-five years or older when they were injured.

Kevin Guskiewicz and his University of North Carolina research team found a higher prevalence of Alzheimer's in NFL players than in the general population, with the difference particularly apparent in people 69 years of age or older. The team found a relatively low overall rate for developing the disease, however: only slightly over 1 percent of former NFL players received a diagnosis of Alzheimer's.

Reviews and meta-analyses (which combine and analyze data from various studies) provide another approach to sort out all the literature and find answers. For example, neurologist David Perry and his UCSF colleagues conducted a meta-analysis of fifty-seven studies to determine the odds of people with a previous TBI developing Alzheimer's, Parkinson's, mild cognitive impairment, or a psychiatric disorder. They uncovered evidence of an association between TBI, including mild TBI, and neurological and psychiatric illness. The authors speculate that there may be some shared characteristics, whether biological or other, to explain this association.

UCSF neurosurgeon Geoffrey Manley and his team reviewed more than 3,800 scientific and medical studies in order to investigate sports-related concussion outcomes. They concluded that the majority of former athletes report their functioning to be similar to that of people in the general population. However, they also concluded that a group of studies showed a relationship between the number of concussions and the rate of depression for retired NFL players and collegiate football players. And they concluded that there is "emerging evidence that some retired athletes have mild cognitive impairment, neuroimaging abnormalities and differences in brain metabolism disproportionate to their age."

But big data research is inconsistent. The International Collaboration on Mild Traumatic Brain Injury Prognosis analyzed the findings from about one hundred studies and failed to find an association between mild TBI and dementia. Internist Paul Crane and his University of Washington colleagues also found no association between

TBI and dementia, or probable Alzheimer's, in participants sixty-five years or older who had a history of TBI that included loss of consciousness. A Finnish team of researchers led by Leena Himanen also found that the particular cognitive problems and patterns of recovery for people with TBI seem to differ from those that characterize Alzheimer's patients.

Other NDs and TBI

Parkinson's disease is an ND that is primarily a movement disorder (with stiff gait and tremor), but Parkinson's can also progress to dementia. Paul Crane's research team found that patients with a history of TBI with a loss of consciousness are at risk for Parkinson's, and those with the most severe TBI incur the greatest risk. These associations remain for a prolonged period following a TBI. However, relatively small numbers of patients in this study actually developed Parkinson's. Raquel Gardner and her team found that a TBI sustained after age 55 is associated with a 40 percent chance of developing Parkinson's within five to seven years. Public health researcher Siavash Jafari and his University of British Columbia colleagues conducted a meta-analysis of twenty-two studies, and they also concluded that there is an increased risk for Parkinson's after a TBI.

Once again, researchers with the International Collaboration on Mild Traumatic Brain Injury Prognosis remained skeptical in their 2014 research review. They concluded that "The best available evidence argues against an important causal association between MTBI and [Parkinson's disease] PD. There are few high-quality studies on this topic. Prospective studies of long duration would address the limitations of recall of head injury and the possibility of reverse causation." Reverse causation means that Parkinson's may have caused the person to be injured, most likely by a fall, rather than that a TBI caused Parkinson's.

ALS also affects movement, because ALS causes motor neurons (neurons that supply the muscles) to degenerate. The disease causes the muscles responsible for moving the arms and legs, breathing, speaking, and swallowing to fail. ALS patients can also experience cognitive and behavioral problems similar to those seen in people with other NDs. Up to 10 percent of ALS cases may be inherited, and in those cases the disease starts earlier on average (age 50, rather than 55 to 65). New York Yankee first baseman Henry Louis Gehrig was 37 when he died of ALS, making it likely that he inherited the disease.

In 1994, the National Institute for Occupational Safety and Health (NIOSH) reported four cases of ALS among NFL players. A subsequent NIOSH study of more than 3,400 NFL football players with at least five years of playing the sport between 1959 and 1988 found the overall risk of death associated with an ND to be three times higher than in the general US population. They found the risk of Alzheimer's and ALS (diagnosed and recorded on death certificates, but not confirmed by autopsy) to be four times higher in this group of football players. However, only seventeen deaths involved one of these diseases, and only ten individuals died from them, so the absolute risk was small, and the group's overall mortality rate was unexpectedly lower than average.

In 2019, Kevin Bieniek and his colleagues at University of Texas / Southwestern found that approximately 6 percent of a group of 300 athletes and 450 nonathletes whose brains were available for study in a brain bank had CTE. American football had the highest frequency of CTE of the sports studied—15 percent—with participation after high school associated with the highest risk.

What Else Might Be a Risk?

What about other disorders of the brain that might be linked to TBI? Epidemiologist Scott Montgomery and his colleagues conducted an observational study using large Swedish databases and a case-control method to study the risk of multiple sclerosis (MS), an immune-mediated disease of the brain and spinal cord. Multiple sclerosis is typically diagnosed in people aged 20 to 40, with triggers even earlier, and with genetic and environmental factors at play. Environmental factors may include ultraviolet light, Vitamin D and Vitamin A, smoking, viruses such as the Epstein-Barr virus, which causes mononucleosis, factors related to the microbiome (gut bacteria), and trauma.

These MS researchers studied young people—children, ages 0 to 10, and adolescents, ages 11 to 20—and speculated that a concussion may cause neuroinflammation and an auto-immune attack on myelin in some young people as they reach adulthood. For every subject with MS after age 20, the researchers found ten subjects without MS—matched in terms of age, sex, geographic area or residence, and then matched with another set of subjects. They found an increased risk of MS for adolescents with a history of concussion, but not for younger children, with a higher risk if the adolescent had had more than one concussion. The researchers also looked at a group of children and adolescents who had fractures (but no concussions) and did not find an increased risk of MS for these young people. Canadian researcher Carole Lunny and her colleagues conducted a meta-analysis of MS and TBI and concluded, however, that much more research is needed to explore the associations between TBI and MS.

Researchers have also raised questions about possible other risks—for stroke and brain tumors. Taiwanese researcher Shih-Wei Liu and colleagues conducted a nationwide study of the risk of stroke after TBI and found that even one concussion significantly raises the risk of ischemic or hemorrhagic stroke. Southern California epidemiologist Susan Preston-Martin and her colleagues found a higher than average risk of brain tumors, particularly meningiomas in men, among people with a history of TBI. The risk correlated more with those who had played collision sports, who were diagnosed with tumors many years following a TBI. Yi-Hua Chen and her colleagues at Taipei Medical University found an increased risk of malignant tumors in a group of patients followed for three years after a TBI. However, UK neurosurgeons Matthew Kirkman and Angelique Albert rightfully raised questions about drawing conclusions, given the small numbers of patients with a tumor diagnosis and some concerns about the research design.

Lingering Questions

Steroids, performance-enhancing drugs, and alcohol consumption need to be added to the list of variables suspected of contributing to NDs, although these factors are harder to investigate because they depend on subjects accurately reporting their substance use. TBI itself is associated with greater risks of mental health disorders and addiction. Neurosurgeon and Steelers' physician Joseph Maroon and his University of Pittsburgh co-authors reviewed the literature and reported that approximately 20 percent of all pathologically confirmed CTE cases (a cohort of about 150 athletes and others) came with a documented history of exposure to substances such as androgenic-anabolic steroids (AASs), alcohol, methamphetamines, cocaine, prescription pain-killers (opioids or opiates), and marijuana, prior to or concurrent with CTE symptoms.

Athletes use AASs, synthetic derivatives of testosterone, to improve muscle strength, endurance, and power, to increase lean body mass, and to enhance recovery between workouts and after an injury. Chronic AAS use is associated with increased aggression, depression, mood and anxiety disorders, irritability, and suicidal tendencies. Weight gain and testicular atrophy (shrinking of the testes) can also occur with AAS use. Canadian researcher Dhananjay Namjoshi and his colleagues showed the cellular effects of repetitive concussion in mice that are also exposed to AAS: white matter (axonal) loss and gliosis.

The Football Players Health Study researchers at Harvard University published early results of their analysis of 3,400 former players. They found that the players who sustained more concussion symptoms during their football years were more likely to report erectile dysfunction later in life and to have low testosterone. Other conditions such as sleep apnea, hypertension, obesity and prescription pain medication use increased their risk of erectile dysfunction. This is evidence of the multiple factors playing a role in the long-term health of professional football players.

A former tight end for the New England Patriots, Aaron Hernandez, died in prison in April 2017 at the age of 27, of suicide by hanging. When the *New York Times* published the news of Hernandez's death in 2017, journalist Ken Belson reported: "For years, Mr. Hernandez was held up as a particularly egregious example of N.F.L. players running amok off the field." Hernandez played football during his youth in Connecticut and later at the University of Florida, where he failed drug tests and got into a bar fight—possible explanations for why he was only a fourth-round draft pick in 2010. He signed a seven-year, $40 million contract with the New England Patriots prior to the 2012 season. Three years later, Hernandez was convicted of murdering Odin Lloyd, a semi-professional football player who was dating his fiancée's sister. While serving a life sentence for Lloyd's murder, he was accused of a 2012 double murder in Boston. Although acquitted of these earlier murders, he received a sentence of four to five years for gun possession handed down just before his highly controversial death.

After Ann McKee examined Hernandez's brain, she reported Stage 3 CTE—the most severe findings of the disease she had ever seen in a person so young (see Figure 7.) Accounts of athletes and others with CTE are often complicated, as are the lives of most people. Hernandez's brother Jonathan makes that clear in his 2018 book, *The Truth About Aaron: My Journey to Understand My Brother.* Hernandez had early athletic success and won the Pop Warner Inspiration to Youth Award. But a mix of football, drugs, interpersonal struggles, conflicts over his sexual orientation, and violence off the field complicated his life, and all these factors interconnect in his story. However, in Aaron Hernandez's case, the graphic images of his destroyed brain make clear that brain damage played a crucial role in the derailment that led to his downward spiral and ultimate death.

Courtroom Science

In 2011, a group of NFL players sued the league, seeking medical and other benefits for those who had contracted certain NDs. The players charged that the NFL had known about but hid evidence of concussion's dangers. They reached a settlement in 2017 when the league agreed to pay affected players over sixty-five years, with $675 million set aside to earn interest over the life of the settlement.

Eligible retired NFL football players can undergo baseline neuropsychological and neurological examinations and additional testing, counseling, and treatment if they qualify. To qualify, they must be diagnosed with moderate cognitive impairment. The settlement includes monetary awards for diagnoses of death with CTE before April 22, 2015, or for those living with ALS, Parkinson's disease, Alzheimer's disease, and other moderate or early dementias. Most who file claims will be players who received diagnoses of dementia, including Alzheimer's, the disease with the highest occurrence rate. Predictions are that the highest awards, however, will go to people with Parkinson's, ALS, or CTE. But Mike Webster's family, for example, may not receive any money, because Webster's death precedes the court's cutoff date. Ken Belson of the *New York Times* reported in 2018 that a provision in the legal settlement could prevent players such as Webster, who died before 2006, from receiving compensation. Some NFL players or their families have chosen not to register for this settlement. Other NFL players are deciding to leave the sport behind altogether. In 2014, Chris Borland, a star rookie for the San Francisco 49ers, bowed out of his profession, citing the sport's dangers, and others, such as Andrew Luck, quarterback for the Indianapolis Colts, have followed his example.

More evidence about repeat concussions and CTE continues to accumulate. Gil Rabinovici, a neurologist and researcher at UCSF, sums up the research this way: "as knowledge of the disorder [CTE] increases, a relationship that is not founded on cause and effect becomes increasingly implausible." Research to date strongly argues for limiting our exposure to brain impacts, and this research implicates all combat and collision sports and affects all age groups.

Bigger than the NFL

In the United States and across the globe, athletes and their representatives are beginning to engage in legal actions similar to the one case that players filed against the NFL. In 2018, the National Hockey League (NHL) settled a case for $19 million with hundreds of retired players who sued the league for hiding the dangers of concussion. Although this was a much lower amount than the NFL settlement, it is another example of what is to come from the legal world for collision sports. The NCAA and college football conferences such as the Big Ten face a group of lawsuits. Plaintiffs charge organizations and academic institutions with failing to protect the health and safety of athletes and fraudulently concealing the dangers of football. There is also growing evidence that other athletes, not just football players, have an increased risk of NDs. In an Italian study of more than 7,000 former professional soccer players, researchers identified the risk of ALS at approximately six times higher than expected for the general population.

Actually, relatively few athletes play professional or even collegiate collision sports. For example, fewer than 2,000 men play in the NFL, approximately 70,000 men play college football, and about 80,000 men and women play college soccer. On the other hand, staggering numbers of children, youth, and young adults participate in organized sports. More than 44 million youth and approximately half of all US high school students play an organized sport. In 1991, a study based on the National Health Interview Survey estimated the annual incidence of sports and recreational concussions in the United States as 1.6 to 3.8 million. The survey's researchers had to use estimates of concussions without loss of consciousness because of how concussion codes worked during this period, and they then inflated the figure to compensate. More recently, University of Washington epidemiologist Mersine Bryan and her research collaborators used multiple databases to produce an annual estimate of 1.1 to 1.9 million concussions for adolescents and children ages 18 or under.

More than a quarter of a million children and youth ages 5 to 14 play football. More than 1 million high school athletes play football, and more than 1 million play soccer or lacrosse, other collision sports with high rates of concussion. Hundreds of thousands of other children, adolescents, and young adults participate in basketball, cheerleading, gymnastics, wrestling, water polo, martial arts, baseball, softball, and other sports with high concussion risks. We should not forget that Ann McKee's brain bank studies have identified CTE in young athletes playing a variety of sports, not just football.

Science, Medicine, and Insurance

The scientific understanding of concussion continues to evolve as research inevitably moves forward. But because we still do not know how to predict whether or when an individual will ultimately fall prey to one of these disorders, the medical community's most important obligation is to warn people with repetitive concussions that they face a significant risk. This warning is just as important as warnings about the health risks of other unhealthy activities, such as smoking. Parents and children, adolescents and young adults, and adults who participate in youth, school, collegiate, and professional sports or other activities that put them at risk for repetitive concussions must each decide for themselves whether to participate.

The latest and possibly the greatest threat to the survival of the NFL and all collision sports is an insurance crisis. ESPN reporters Steve Fainaru and Mark Fainaru-Wada write that the NFL no longer has general liability insurance covering head trauma, and only one insurance carrier is willing to provide workers' compensation coverage for NFL teams. They put it this way: "To an increasing number of carriers, football is a dam built atop an earthquake fault. A disaster might never occur, but the specter of huge potential losses is scaring many companies away." ESPN's television program *Outside the Lines* conducted interviews of carriers, brokers, lawyers, athletic officials, school administrators, and athletes. The results suggest that youth football, and possibly other collision sports, are now caught up in this insurance crisis. Some schools are opting out of football and other high-risk sports. With apologies to Hamlet: To play or not to play, that is the question—a question to be explored further in Part Two.

Part Two

To Play or Not to Play

Historically most concussions were not considered serious, and athletes who sustained them might be said to have been "dinged" or had their "bell rung."¹ The injured player would "shake it off" and return to play. . . . Culture is created by the sum of beliefs and behaviors within a group . . . it is clear to us that currently, in many settings, the seriousness of the threat to the health of an athlete, both acute and long term, from suffering a concussion is not fully appreciated or acted upon.

—THE INSTITUTE OF MEDICINE AND
THE NATIONAL RESEARCH COUNCIL, 2014

5

Exercising Sensibly

THE BENEFITS OF exercise have been extolled for millennia. Thomas Jefferson wrote: "Leave all the afternoon for exercise and recreation, which are as necessary as reading. I will rather say more necessary because health is worth more than learning." Yet a paradox lies in wait: exercise has clear benefits, but it also entails the risk of injury. The good news is that we can reduce certain risks for concussions and other injuries in our leisure activities. Deciding whether and how to exercise entails calculating the risk-benefit ratio, but top fitness, education and training, adherence to safety precautions, the highest quality equipment, and the best environmental conditions can mitigate the risk. The mechanisms or methods that reduce injury risk define primary prevention. More people engage in recreational activities than team sports (the focus of Chapter 6), so we must address exercise and play in these activities. Not every concussion can be avoided, but most can be prevented.

Bicycles

Given all the media attention the sport receives, you might think football tops the sports and recreational injury list for emergency rooms (ERs) across the United States. But that's not the case. That distinction goes to bicycling, an activity about which Mark Twain cautioned, with his typical sense of irony: "Get a bicycle. You will not regret it, if you live."

In fact, bicycle-related injuries produce more than half a million ER visits each year in the United States. The US Consumer Product Safety Commission uses a tracking system called the National Electronic Injury Surveillance System (NEISS) to track product-related injuries. The American Association of Neurological Surgeons, using NEISS data, estimates that bicycle crashes play a role in about one of every five sports- and recreation-related traumatic brain injuries (TBIs) treated in ERs. In comparison, football accounts for about one in ten ER visits. More than 70 percent of all children between the ages of 5 and 14 ride bicycles, many more than the number who play football. For children under age 14, cycling causes almost double the number of ER cases involving a concussion or more serious TBI compared to football. Cycling is also a far more gender-neutral sport than football, and its participants span a broader age range. Cycling injuries affect people of all ages and as many women and girls as men and boys.

Bicycling in the United States and in many other countries around the world is a growth industry, fueled by factors such as rising gasoline prices, lower likelihood of car ownership among the young, greater availability of paths and lanes for bicycles, and a rising interest in bicycling for commuting as well as for pleasure. Bike-share or bike-hire programs have cropped up in cities across the world. Cycling events raise money for charities, and competitive cycling is on the rise.

With this growth comes increased numbers of injuries and deaths. Thomas Sanford and colleagues at the University of California San Francisco (UCSF) found a troubling increase in bicycle injuries when they analyzed data from 100 emergency departments in the United States between 1998 and 2013. Injuries rose 28 percent, and ensuing hospitalizations increased 120 percent, with the greatest rise for people over age 45. The percentage of cyclists with head injuries rose from 10 percent to 16 percent over this time period. Street bicycle injuries, which are likely to involve cars, also increased. While many bicycle mishaps occur without involving another vehicle, cyclists are at especially high risk of colliding with heavier motor vehicles.

During the 1990s, biking was primarily an activity of the young in the United States. In decades past, it was rare for anyone over age 55 to ride a bicycle, and almost unheard of for anyone over age 75 to do so. A rapid drop in car use among young adults might suggest that millennials have been driving the nationwide cycling boom, but the increase in cyclists from 1995–2009 actually reveals a new generational trend. The National Household Travel Survey authors report that bike usage by people aged 60 to 79 in the United States accounted for more than one-third of the total increase in bike trips from 1995–2009, which is the largest percentage increase of any group.

Most cycling fatalities occur not at intersections, as one might think, but on streets and roadways. Streets that have dedicated bike lanes see many fewer crashes that result in death or serious injury. Bike paths or lanes painted a different color may help to prevent crashes, but a completely separate surface, divided from the street or roadway by a barrier, is the ideal.

Cyclists riding on streets should ride in the same direction as cars and be visible to them. Learning and obeying the rules of the road is essential for cyclists and drivers alike, and that includes proper signaling, stopping, and respecting others, including pedestrians. Drivers must be respectful of cyclists and give them ample room. Checking the rearview mirrors before exiting a vehicle to make sure a cyclist is not riding by can prevent injuries, not just to cyclists but also to other drivers and their passengers. One study found that car doors opening into traffic caused about one-third of bicycle crashes.

The Netherlands, a country with more than 22 million bicycles (1.3 per capita) enacted a rule in 2016, informally called "The Dutch Reach," requiring drivers to use their right hand to open their vehicle's door, making it more likely that they will spot a cyclist pulling up next to the car as they turn. *New York Times* journalist Tanya Mohn thinks the United States should adopt this rule, too. A severe brain injury might have been prevented in one of my patients who was getting out of the driver's seat of her car as a cyclist was passing.

A bicycle should fit its rider well and be well-maintained for safe operation. A child or adult should be able to straddle the bike with both feet on the ground. Young children need bicycles with coaster brakes until they can squeeze brake levers on handlebars. Bikes must have good lighting in front, sufficient to be seen 300 feet ahead. A red reflector should be visible from 500 feet behind the bicycle, and reflectors on the pedals should be visible at 200 feet. A handlebar or helmet mirror enables a rider to spot vehicle activity from behind. A bell or horn alerts pedestrians when necessary. Cyclists should always wear bright clothing or reflecting materials that are clearly visible at a distance. Children and adults should wear clothing that will not get caught in spokes or chains, as well as shoes rather than sandals or flip-flops. Clip pedals help racers go faster, but for noncompetitive riders, they pose the danger of catching a foot and causing a fall if the cyclist needs to stop suddenly or dismount quickly.

We teach very few children and adults how to safely ride a bicycle or use other wheeled devices. Most of us learn by the seat of our pants. Experts advise that we should be trained to ride just as we are trained to drive. Schools and police departments offer lessons in some communities. Until age 10, children can ride bikes on sidewalks, but usually not beyond that age in many areas of the country. Once riders begin to cycle on hills and winding roads, they may require more detailed and specific instruction and training. For example, riders can prevent falls by learning to carry most of their body weight on the feet and pedals, rather than the hands and handlebars, and by keeping the outside pedal down when they take a curve. Given higher rates of unsafe driving and cycling in older age groups, fitness evaluations and additional skills training might reduce injury and death rates.

Half of children ages 5 to 14 in the United States own a helmet, according to Safe Kids Worldwide. Unfortunately, only about one-quarter report always wearing it while bicycling. (The CDC reports a much lower figure—just 15 percent.) Using a helmet will not prevent a concussion, but it can limit the severity of an injury. Eight states and the District of Columbia require children to wear a helmet while riding wheeled vehicles such as scooters, skateboards, or in-line skates. The Consumer Product Safety Commission has created standards for manufacturing and using helmets. The helmet should cover the forehead, sit horizontally, not tilt toward the back of the head, and be secured by snug chin straps. Riders should replace their helmet periodically with a new one that carries the highest rating, fits properly, covers the forehead, and has diamond-shaped straps around the ears that securely fasten under the chin.

Recall that Jason, the ER physician introduced in Chapter 1, wore a top-notch helmet that absorbed much of the force applied to his head when he catapulted from his bike. The helmet did not prevent his concussion, but had he not been wearing it, his injury would have been far worse. Just as with football helmets, bicycle helmets mostly protect against skull fractures and more serious TBIs. When bicycle riders do not wear helmets, crashes frequently result in serious TBIs or death. Nine out of ten bicyclists killed in the United States are not wearing helmets and, notably, a majority of these riders are middle-aged men.

Across the world, bicycles now number about one billion. Mandatory helmet laws exist in Australia, Canada, the Czech Republic, Finland, Iceland, New Zealand, and Sweden. In the United States, these laws vary from state to state. Some countries do not have helmet laws because of prevailing opinions that helmets give riders a false sense of safety and that other preventive measures are more important. During the boom in cycling in Europe that began in the mid-1970s, cycling injuries and fatalities declined dramatically in Germany and the Netherlands, most likely because of changes in infrastructure, public awareness, and education. While the worldwide helmet debate for cyclists will likely continue, statistics suggest that helmets are critical safety factors for US children and adults engaged in any wheeled activity, self-propelled or motorized.

Other Wheeled Equipment

Bicycle injury incidence is especially high because there are so many cyclists. But other wheeled equipment—wagons, tricycles, mopeds and minibikes, roller and in-line skates, skateboards, longboards, and scooters—also plays a role in many injuries and deaths each year. Motorized recreational conveyances such as all-terrain vehicles (ATVs), dune buggies, go-carts, motorized scooters, hoverboards, and self-balancing personal transporters such as the Segway can create dangers for their riders and pedestrians. Speed, safety features, reliability, rider ability, and terrain all factor into the level of risk.

The newer electric self-balancing scooters (ESSs) introduced to streets and roadways in urban America and in other countries present a rising risk of injury. ESS proponents argue that the vehicles are environmentally friendly, provide efficient ways to navigate for short distances, and may spur road safety initiatives such as bike lane development. But statistics have been accumulating regarding rider injury risks, including concussion and more serious brain injuries. Injuries to pedestrians are a concern as well. Scooter companies do not provide or make helmets available, and most riders do not wear them. Tarak Trivedi and colleagues at the University of California Los Angeles (UCLA) examined the ER records of 249 injured patients and raised red flags about this risky new mode of transportation. About 10 percent of patients were younger than 18, the minimum age permitted by scooter companies. Only ten of the 249 were wearing a helmet. It's not surprising that 40 percent of those injured had head injuries.

Equestrian Sports

Wheeled devices aren't the only contributor to ER statistics. In a multi-center study using a trauma database, Ethan Winkler and fellow UCSF researchers investigated sports-related TBIs diagnosed in ERs across five sports categories (roller sports, skiing / snowboarding, equestrian sports, and aquatic sports). Equestrian sports represented 45 percent of these injuries.

Many horseback riders fall on their heads, either catapulting forward as actor Christopher Reeve did, sliding sideways off the horse, or being kicked by the horse after they fall. Riders aged 10 to 14 are the most likely to be involved in an accident with a horse, and more than half of those injured are girls. Anyone who has mounted a horse knows that height off the ground factors heavily in equestrian injury rates. An inexperienced rider, a skittish horse, slippery terrain, or riding bareback are factors that may increase the risk of falling.

Judy, my patient whose injury was described in Chapter 2, wasn't wearing a helmet when her horse threw her. Most recreational or Western equestrians do not wear helmets, which are required for English riding events and equestrian sports that involve jumping and high-level dressage competitions. But English riders also often wear top hats, which provide no protection at all, and many riders do not wear helmets when they practice for competitions that require helmets. Rodeo riders have begun turning in their cowboy hats for helmets, and they offer good advice about falling for other riders—tuck your chin and use your arms to protect your head. Cyclists and other wheeled riders can also benefit from this advice.

Snow and Ice

Skiing and snowboarding are the most popular winter sports in the United States, with 10 million participants each year. About 600,000 people annually incur injuries while engaging in these sports, and one in five of these injuries involves a TBI, which is also the injury most likely to cause death or disability for skiers. Recreational skiers and snowboarders can reach speeds of over forty miles per hour. According to the National Ski Areas Association (NSAA) 2012–2013 National Demographic Study, about seven out of ten skiers and snowboarders wear helmets. As is the case with bicycling, a helmet does not completely protect against injury when a skier hits a tree or lands hard on the ground, but it may limit the severity of an injury. Actor and politician Sonny Bono and actress Natasha Richardson both suffered fatal TBIs while skiing. Neither wore a helmet. For good reason, more and more skiers are adding helmets to their ski gear.

The NSAA "Lids on Kids" program and other helmet promotion programs may be having a positive effect, because the use of helmets has been rising among downhill skiers. Cross-country skiing does not carry the same risk as downhill skiing. Although cross-country skiers fall, they do not reach anywhere near the speeds of downhill skiers. Thus helmets are not required for recreational cross-country skiers. Other winter sports—sledding, snowboarding, snow tubing, ice skating, and ice hockey—also carry risks of concussion, especially for young and novice participants. The US Consumer Product Safety Commission provides the best reference for help deciding which helmet to choose for each winter sport.

The Extremes

The idea of extreme sports calls to mind humorist Erma Bombeck's quip about not participating in any sport with ambulances at the bottom of the hill. Enthusiasm for these supremely fit and talented risk-takers has been fueled by dedicated TV channels, internet sites, and media coverage of the Olympics and Paralympics. These sports include alpine skiing, ski jumping, snowboarding, all-terrain vehicle (ATV) sports, bicycle motor cross (BMX), bungee jumping, hang gliding/paragliding, mountaineering, mountain biking, skydiving, and surfing and involve elite athletes, high speeds and heights, extreme levels of physical exertion, elaborate stunts, and real dangers to participants, even those who are highly skilled. The highest risks occur in alpine skiing and surfing.

The International Ski Federation (FIS) is the international governing body for winter sports. The organization studied alpine, freestyle, snowboarding, ski jumping, and cross-country events from 2006 to 2018 and reported that about 11 percent of the 3,554 injuries involved concussions or other neurological conditions. Athletes who run the aerials course most fear the snapping back of the head and neck against the snow, referred to as a "slap back," which can lead to severe brain and spinal cord injuries.

Olympian Elana Meyers Taylor and other bobsledders soar down icy paths at breakneck speeds of up to 90 miles per hour. Meyers Taylor took a spill at the end of one descent at the Winter Olympics in Sochi, Russia, and landed on her head. Despite her accident, she won the silver medal in Sochi and won again in the 2018 Winter Olympics in PyeongChang, South Korea, competing in luge. After the Sochi Olympics, she underwent a prolonged recovery for a concussion, and she reports that she had suffered other concussions. Meyers Taylor has announced publicly that she is donating her brain for science and the study of chronic traumatic encephalopathy (CTE). She pleads for more women winter athletes to follow her lead by donating their brains to research.

For the para or adapted sports athlete (an athlete with a disability), the topic of concussion is just beginning to emerge in the scientific and clinical literature. Editors Yetsa Tuakli-Wosorno and Wayne Derman tackled the topic in an issue of *Physical Medicine and Rehabilitation Clinics of North America* in 2018. Para athletes are exposed to concussion risk, just as are other athletes in speed, collision, and contact sports, but concussion assessment, management, and risk reduction strategies must be adapted for these athletes because they face somewhat different risks.

There are relatively few people, with or without disabilities, who have the desire and the skills to participate in professional extreme sports, but many amateur or recreational athletes take risks that are incompatible with their skill levels. We don't have statistics on this, only anecdotes. I clearly remember patients in this category.

Most regretted their decisions to try daredevil stunts on ATVs, skateboards, or skis, for example. These athletes might find as much fun with considerably less risk (but not necessarily no risk) on playgrounds and at gyms.

Playgrounds and Gyms

According to the Centers for Disease Control and Prevention (CDC), falls cause more than half of the TBIs among children ages 14 and younger, and many occur on playgrounds or in backyards. In 2013, ERs in the United States treated more than 29,000 children for playground concussions and other serious head injuries, up from 18,000 in 2001. About two-thirds of these injuries occurred at schools and recreational sports facilities. Sixty percent of these ER patients were boys, and more than half were aged 5 to 9. One out of three ER visits in the 5 to 9 age group involved monkey bars, and a quarter involved swings, while swings or slides were the more likely culprits for children 4 and under.

Sarah, the patient I treated as an adult, had fallen backward from a swing when she was 4 years old and suffered a concussion that triggered a seizure (see Chapter 2). Sarah's mother, a nurse, knew that keeping kids out of harm's way required an ongoing balancing act between fun, exercise, fresh air, peer pressure (what "all the other kids" are doing), and common sense. Sarah was just at the age when she might have been considered old enough to use a full-size swing. But her mother was watching from the park bench, and Sarah wasn't holding on tightly enough when she fell backward on the packed-earth surface of the playground. A safer surface with loosely packed material such as rubber might have prevented or lessened Sarah's injury.

Playground injuries occur for many reasons. Children may be too young to use certain equipment. They may be inadequately supervised, or other children may pressure them to participate in activities they are not ready for. Helmets, so useful for bike riding, skating, and skateboarding, provide no solution on the playground or at the park because they may make climbing unsafe. Pediatricians can advise about age-appropriate playground use, and some playgrounds post age or height requirements, warnings, and advice for those supervising children.

Another leisure-time activity, trampoline use, continues to grow in popularity despite more and more injuries to children and youth in backyards and parks across the United States. Falls on or off a trampoline, impact with a trampoline frame or springs, flips and somersaults gone awry, or users colliding with one another while jumping can cause neck, head, and other injuries. The majority of these injuries occur in backyards, but trampoline parks have become a billion-dollar business. As the trampoline industry grows, the number of injuries has spiked. Kathryn Kasmire of Connecticut Children's Medical Center and her colleagues reported the increase in 2016: US emergency department visits for trampoline park injuries increased from 581 in 2010 to 6,932 in 2014, whereas home trampoline injuries did not increase during that time period.

Indoor gym environments can also house injury risks for adults, youth, and children beyond simple muscle sprains and strains. Home gyms may seem to be a safe place to work out and get the health benefits of exercise without having to pay to join a gym or health club and travel to exercise, but some injuries occur at home. Hospital ERs treat about half a million injuries involving exercise equipment annually, according to the US Consumer Product Safety Commission. Usually the problem involves operator failure rather than faulty equipment. This means that individual choices—getting proper instruction and developing fitness to participate in the activity—are key to preventing injury.

Treadmills, for example, carry a risk of concussion and more severe TBIs, as we learned in 2015 from the death of businessman Dave Goldberg, former CEO of Survey Monkey and husband of Facebook COO Sheryl Sandberg. Goldberg had a cardiac arrhythmia that caused him to fall off a treadmill, and in the fall, he suffered the TBI that contributed to his death. Treadmills can be dangerous for those who fall and have no one to assist them or to call 911 if necessary. Without an attached safety clip that triggers the machine to stop when detached, the treadmill keeps moving, causing further injury. Other equipment may be positioned too close to the treadmill, creating a hazard for someone who falls. There should be a minimum of six feet without obstructions behind a treadmill.

Get Up and Go

The bottom line is that while we should strive to be physically active, we also need to be educated and cautious. We can dramatically reduce our risk by using good judgment, the highest quality equipment, and safe practices as we exercise and play during our leisure time. Developing and then maintaining the requisite physical and mental fitness for a particular recreational activity is critical. There are many ways to enjoy safe, health-promoting, and otherwise rewarding exercise that carries very little, if any, concussion risk.

6

Game Changers

N OCTOBER 2006, 13-year-old Zackery Lystedt fell while tackling an opposing player in a junior varsity football game in Tacoma, Washington. He landed hard on the turf, receiving a severe blow to the head. His coach sidelined him, but Zack returned to the game in the second half. As the game ended, Zack collapsed, unconscious. Airlifted to Harborview Medical Center, Zach remained in a coma. He emerged from coma after three months, but he continues to have difficulty speaking clearly, remembering, and walking.

Zack and his parents and other advocates pushed for Washington State to enact the Zackery Lystedt Law, a comprehensive statute to protect youth athletes, which passed in 2009. Zack and his family lobbied for laws across the United States, and now every state has enacted at least some type of concussion legislation. Yet despite increased concussion awareness and changes in legislation, other tragedies have occurred across the country, including in the state of Washington. In 2015, Kenney Bui, a star pupil with a passion for football, died from a severe brain injury incurred during a high school game in Tacoma. Like Zack, Kenney had also been cleared to play after suffering a concussion earlier in the season.

In 2013, reporter Thomas Zambito interviewed the family of deceased junior varsity football player Ryne Dougherty of Montclair, New Jersey, following the family's legal settlement with the Montclair School District. Before boarding the team bus for a game in the fall of 2008, the 16-year-old told his stepfather, "Today is my game and I'm gonna be a star." During that game, Ryne was hit hard in a tackle, and he suffered what appeared to be a concussion followed by a seizure on the field. According to news reports, he stood up, answered some questions from his trainers, then collapsed as he walked to the sidelines. He remained in a coma until he died two days later from a brain hemorrhage. A few weeks earlier during a practice, Ryne had suffered another injury that appeared to be a concussion. According to news reports, even though Ryne continued to experience headaches and blurred vision, his family physician cleared him to return to football. The family's lawyer later argued that the school had violated its own guidelines, permitting Ryne to play despite his ongoing symptoms. The family eventually settled a lawsuit against Ryne's school and their township's Board of Education for $2.8 million.

Young athletes like Zack, Kenney, and Ryne are more likely to be seriously injured playing collision sports than older athletes. The injuries these boys suffered are referred to as second-impact syndrome (SIS). Coined in 1984, the term refers to a devastating second brain injury that occurs in an athlete who has had symptoms or signs suggesting a brain injury and then suffers a catastrophic second injury. One theory is that the immature brain fits more tightly within the skull and contains a higher concentration of water than the mature brain. The second concussion or more serious brain injury disrupts cerebral blood flow, and rapid and catastrophic swelling of the brain ensues. The second injury may follow the first within hours, days, or weeks. We don't know how severe the first brain injuries were for Zack, Kenney, or Ryne because no imaging studies were obtained on any of these boys until the devastating events occurred.

Joseph Chernach played football from the age of 11 to 14. After he committed suicide when he was 22 years old, Ann McKee's lab at Boston University found evidence of chronic traumatic encephalopathy (CTE) in his post-mortem brain. Ken Belson recounted the story in the *New York Times* in 2016. Chernach's family filed a suit against Pop Warner, the nation's largest youth football league, and settled in 2016 for an undisclosed amount. Another class action lawsuit represents every current and former Pop Warner player since 1997 and contends that Pop Warner, the National Operating Committee on Standards for Athletic Equipment (NOCSAE), and USA Football (an organization for youth football funded by the NFL) failed to uphold their duties to provide for the safety and health of child athletes, misleading and deceiving parents and children about football's risks to the human brain.

These tragic stories link brain injuries during collision sports play to the direst outcomes. Because these catastrophic outcomes happen rarely, we have no large populations to study, so the prevalence and predictors of SIS and CTE in young people remain unknown. Nevertheless, tragedies such as these must impel us to prevent other catastrophic injuries.

Not Just SIS and CTE

Concussions in young athletes such as those experienced by Carla, who played soccer in high school, and Tom, a college football player, are much more common than the concussions suffered by Zack, Kenney, Ryne, or Joseph, but they are still worrisome. Both Carla and Tom suffered more than one concussion and ongoing symptoms. Tom did not completely recover, likely because he had had so many concussions over the years. He never returned to the football field or college but was able to get vocational training in carpentry. Carla eventually recovered, and she went on to college with an athletic scholarship.

Thomas Dompier, an athletic trainer and professor at Lebanon Valley College, undertook a large-scale review of concussion incidence during the 2012 and 2013 football seasons with his other colleagues. They found that 1 in 30 youth football players, 1 in 14 high school players, and 1 in 20 college players sustained one or more concussions. Many suffered more than one. Once an athlete has a first concussion, the risk of another occurring seems to increase. For example, University of Michigan researcher Eric Zemper showed the risk of another concussion in concussed high school and college football players to be almost six times greater than those players without a history of concussion. Concussions also raise the odds of other injuries after return to play, as Illinois State University researcher Robert Lynall and colleagues found in a study of college athletes. Anna Nordström and her colleagues in Sweden found that one concussion increases the risk of subsequent injury by about 50 percent in male elite football teams in ten European countries.

Recurrent concussions also increase the risk of persistent symptoms that can linger and affect school, work, or life in general for days, months, or even years in some people. Psychologist Danielle Ransom and her colleagues analyzed the effects of post-concussion symptoms on academic performance for students in elementary, middle, and high school for more than 300 students ages 5 to 18 who had sustained a concussion. The students completed questionnaires within four weeks of their injury. Those who had more symptoms were more likely to report problems at school. The more severe the symptoms, the more they correlated with the total number of academic problems students and parents reported, regardless of how much time had passed since the student's injury.

Nearly 90 percent of the students in Ransom's study reported at least one problem, such as headache, fatigue, or problems concentrating, while about 75 percent reported such problems as trouble taking notes, needing a longer time to complete homework, and difficulties concentrating. More than 40 percent of participating students reported academic difficulties, even if they no longer had symptoms. This study suggests serious risks from concussion for the developing brain.

Age, Birth Sex, and Gender

Children now tend to play one sport more intensively at younger ages than in the past. In states such as California and Florida, where temperate weather provides more opportunities for outdoor pursuits, sports are often played in three seasons. Relentless exposure to one sport (as opposed to what is called sports sampling) puts student athletes at risk for more injuries, including concussions. Sports specialization has also been linked to shorter careers and a reduced likelihood of success at a sport.

Canadian researcher Francois Gallant and his colleagues found that specializing in one sport prior to adolescence, as compared with sports sampling, resulted in decreased sports participation during adolescence. Pediatrician Joel Brenner and the American Academy of Pediatrics (AAP) strongly recommend waiting until age 15 or 16 (puberty) to specialize in a sport because of this increased injury risk. The organization recommends resting from a specific sports activity one to two days per week. It also supports

taking at least three months off during the year, in one-month in-
crements, from the sport.

Boston University researchers Michael Alosco, Julie Stamm,
and colleagues have published several research studies that support
their hypothesis that the age children start playing football is one
determinant of risk for late-life cognitive problems. These researchers are exploring what is called "the age of first exposure" to
a sport. They tested former NFL players who started playing football before age 12 and found more cognitive problems later in life
in these players than in those who began tackle football when they
were older. In one of this group's studies, MRI scans revealed
more changes in the corpus callosum's white matter tracts in the
group that had participated in football at an earlier age. In a related
study, University of Georgia researcher Julianne Schmidt and co-
investigators found that the age at which an athlete or military
cadet has a first concussion influences the number of subsequent
concussions. These data support the hypothesis that the number of
concussions over an athletic career may make a major difference in
outcomes.

It is difficult to draw conclusions about whether birth sex and
gender play a role in concussion from the few individual stories I have
related here. Both Carla, playing high school soccer, and Tom, playing
college football, experienced severe headaches and serious academic
difficulties after concussions. However, more than one research study
has suggested that girls may suffer more concussions and may have
more severe or prolonged post-concussion symptoms than boys
playing the same sports (such as soccer, basketball, softball or baseball,
and lacrosse). For example, concussion rates are four times higher for
girls playing softball than for boys playing baseball. In some studies,
female athletes report a greater number and greater severity of symptoms after a concussion, require a longer time to recover, and/or

achieve poorer outcomes. One such study by Mount Sinai orthopedist Alexis Colvin and her colleagues found that female soccer players performed worse on the ImPACT and reported more symptoms. If these gender differences are real, are they due to biological, social, or cultural factors?

We can't be certain, but some studies have begun to shed light on a key issue about concussion symptom reporting: boys may be more likely than girls to hide their symptoms because of cultural expectations and how they are socialized to respond or behave. Youngstown State University athletic trainer and researcher Jessica Wallace and her co-investigators found that high school male and female athletes were similarly knowledgeable about concussion, but females were more likely to use that knowledge to report a concussion. In fact, males were four to eleven times more likely than the females to not report a concussion because of "the reactions and perceptions of others."

Researchers speculate about the biological differences related to anatomy or physiology. We know that adolescent males and females differ in cognitive developmental milestones. The size and strength of neck muscles and head-to-soccer-ball size ratios differ, and there may be other differences between female and male athletes who head a soccer ball. In addition to these anatomic and biomechanical differences, males and females differ hormonally. Females experience greater numbers of migraine headaches, and perhaps this explains the increased incidence of post-concussion headaches in girls playing the same sports as boys. There may even be differences in the vulnerability of cellular elements in the brains of females and males, as Jean-Pierre Dollé and his laboratory research colleagues at the University of Pennsylvania have been investigating in animal studies.

Managing Concussion

Olympic and professional contests always include team physicians or athletic trainers on the sidelines. However, this is not necessarily the case with youth, high school, or college practices or games. Unfortunately, even when these professionals are present, reliable concussion decision-making may not occur. All these professionals have both a stake in the sport and in winning games, which raises the question of bias in decisions. This bias can affect decisions about removing an athlete from the field or other determinations that might threaten the welfare of young athletes. Harvard's Emily Kroshus and her research collaborators found evidence of underreporting and pressure from various stakeholders in their study of 328 collegiate athletes from seven different sports in the northeastern United States. More than one-quarter of the athletes had faced pressure from one or more of these stakeholders—a coach, a teammate, a fan, or a parent. In another study, Kroshus found that socioeconomic status was linked to rates of concussion education and certification.

Well-meaning coaches are invested in the success of their student athletes and teams, and they face intense pressure. Schools and coaches may push to increase the numbers of games played and their overall success rate by playing games against poorer performing teams. Running up the scores and numbers of games helps every stakeholder, including youth aspiring to college and college scholarships. Pressure to have unskilled or less skilled student athletes play so they can check the sports participation box on college applications presents another challenge for coaches and trainers. Teachers can make supplemental income coaching. They can also earn a substantial amount of income from work with sports clinics, in addition to regular coaching, if their school districts allow this.

Mayo Clinic physiatrists Katherine Nanos and Edward Las-
kowski investigated how much high school athletes, their coaches,
and parents know about concussions and published their results in
2017. They surveyed 115 athletes, 132 parents, and 15 coaches at
three high schools in Rochester, Minnesota. The athletes played a
variety of sports—football, soccer, volleyball, hockey, basketball,
wrestling, dance, gymnastics, lacrosse, baseball, and softball. The
results were disheartening. Only about one-third of high school
athletes, their coaches, and their parents knew that a concussion is a
brain injury. While most could identify the possible effects of concussion, coaches had the most knowledge about how a concussion
occurs, when to take an athlete out of a game, and the potential effects of repeat head injuries. Athletes were less likely than coaches to
know how a concussion occurs or to understand the criteria for returning to play. Parents who worked in health care had no greater
knowledge about concussions than other parents, yet they had greater
awareness of the long-term effects of concussions, such as chronic
traumatic encephalopathy (CTE).

In 2014, Harvard researcher Christine Baugh and her colleagues
published results of their survey to see if schools had established recommended concussion management plans in response to the policy
and legislation. About 80 percent of schools responded that a plan was
in place. When asked who had the final responsibility for returning
athletes to play after a concussion, the most common responses were
that it was a team physician (80 percent) or athletic trainer (70 percent).
Sometimes it was a specialist physician (30 percent), a coach (7 percent),
or actually the athlete (7 percent). About 75 percent of schools indicated that their institution had a process for annual athlete concussion
education, and about 90 percent required athletes to acknowledge
their responsibility to report concussion symptoms. Although nearly
all respondents thought their school's concussion management plan

protects athletes, many suggested the need for better education pro-grams for coaches, increasing sports medicine staffing, and better athlete education.

Removal and Return to Learn and to Play

When a concussion occurs during an athletic event, the student-athlete should be immediately evaluated by a certified athletic trainer, coach, or licensed health-care professional who will deter-mine what should be done next. Athletes must stop participating or be stopped from participating immediately. They must not return to play the same day, and they must be evaluated by a physician or other licensed health-care provider as soon as possible. Some ath-letes who have injuries to the head through forceful bodily contact, or what are termed "hits," have delayed symptoms—after the game or even over the next day or days, making prompt diagnosis impos-sible. For these athletes, the same protocol must apply once symp-toms occur—no return to play until a physician, or other licensed health-care provider knowledgeable about concussions, completes a diagnostic evaluation and outlines a treatment plan.

University of Arkansas researcher R. J. Elbin and colleagues found that young athletes who continued to play after concussion require nearly twice as long to recover than those who are immedi-ately removed from play (forty-four days versus twenty-two days). In an Ontario study by James Carson and associates using chart re-view as a research method, about 44 percent of students returned to play or to school sooner than symptoms (continuing or worsening) should have dictated. Athletes should not return to playing any sport or participating in any activity that puts them at risk for another concussion, at least until their symptoms have completely resolved, both at rest and with activity. The risk of another concussion is highest within the first ten days, so in many cases, the athlete should remain out of play for at least that amount of time, even if symptoms resolve before ten days. The Berlin International Consensus Statement defines persistent post-concussion symptoms as greater than two weeks for adults and greater than four weeks for children.

Parents are essential to decision-making about return to school and to play because they know their children's medical histories, developmental histories, academic and sports histories, and personalities and habits. The student athlete may want to return to play before their physician recommends it, and they may not disclose symptoms, so parental observation is essential. At a practice or game or afterward, parents may observe a change in personality or mood, such as irritability, anxiety, or depression, or difficulty keeping a schedule and remembering to complete tasks. The student athlete may have difficulty following conversations with more than one person, may avoid situations with overstimulation, experience sensitivity to light and sound, or suffer a change in sleep patterns.

Parents are most likely to be able to tell if their sons and daughters are symptomatic, even if their children deny symptoms to the physician or others in the hopes of getting back on the field. Parents should keep track of recovery with a journal listing symptoms and other problems that arise. Good communication with a daughter or son can help to identify if symptoms continue to be evident. This kind of individualized monitoring is imperative for post-concussion treatment and decisions about when it is possible to return to school or a sport.

Dodging Some Questions

Organizations such as the American Academy of Neurology, the International Conferences on Concussion in Sport, the Ontario Neurotrauma Foundation, the American Medical Society for Sports Medicine, and the Centers for Disease Control (CDC) in collaboration with the American Academy of Pediatrics (AAP) have created sports concussion guidelines and consensus statements over many decades to help physicians and other licensed health-care providers make clinical decisions. These documents attempt to make sense of an unclear and sometimes contradictory area of science and medicine. Clinical and consensus-based guidelines provide treatment recommendations, but they are only recommendations and not recipes for individualized care. In some cases, the guidelines do not address important questions.

The experts producing guidelines and consensus statements now agree that athletes should be removed from play after a concussion and should not return to play the same day. The guidelines also recommend a stepwise reintroduction to exercise, with attention to whether symptoms reappear. But some researchers and clinicians question the entire area of symptom evaluation, including how to determine symptom resolution. The timing for medically clearing athletes to return to play still causes a dilemma because concussion is a condition based primarily on symptoms.

Guideline experts also seem to be avoiding the extremely important topic of repetitive concussions and long-term consequences. We have not yet fully determined whether one concussion is one too many (and for whom), but it has become clear that repeat concussions create a risky set-up for problems later in life, especially for high school and amateur athletes. With each injury, the severity and time of recovery increases, perhaps proof that the brain is more vulnerable and less able to withstand biomechanical forces in the same manner as before an injury.

Past guidelines used a three-concussions rule: an athlete should be retired after three concussions. The experts writing guidelines now say that advice no longer should appear in guidelines because of a lack of research evidence. University of Pennsylvania laboratory researcher Douglas Smith and his co-investigators reviewed the research on repetitive TBIs and concluded that "Current evidence indicates a possible 'dose' and frequency-dependent association between TBI and risk of neurodegenerative disease." In other words, the number of concussions may link to the risk of chronic traumatic encephalopathy (CTE) or another neurodegenerative disease.

Sports medicine researchers Robert Cantu and Johna Register-Mihalik believe that the decision to retire from playing a sport is crucial, and that varying factors contribute to it: "If, with each injury, the severity and length of recovery increases, then a more conservative return or disqualification may be a consideration. The lengthened recovery may be evidence that the brain is more vulnerable and unable to withstand the forces and stresses in the same manner as before the injuries occurred. No specific number of concussions mandates that an individual should definitively be retired from a sport." They go on to state: "Thus, when making return-to-play decisions and, especially, retirement decisions, it is not only important to consider how many prior concussions have been incurred but how many subconcussive impacts have been received based on the sport, position, and style of play." The problem with this advice is that we have no good measures for concussion severity, no good measures of subconcussion, and no good measures of the fuzzy notion of style of play.

These authors state that an athlete should consider retirement if post-concussion symptoms take longer to resolve with each successive injury, if less bodily force is required to produce a concussion, or if imaging studies such as MRI scans demonstrate evidence of brain injury. Unfortunately, a decision to retire from a collision sport using these criteria may occur too late. Such recommendations imply that a young athlete can return to play multiple times before being retired. We must ask: who is counting, or would be able to count, all of the impacts an athlete receives over months and years of playing a collision sport?

Sports medicine researcher Cecilia Davis-Hayes and her colleagues propose an algorithm to assist with retirement from sport decisions, based on reviewing clinical cases. In this guideline, the athlete and parents make this personal decision. They pose these questions as relevant: Is the sport a collision or contact sport? Is the risk for concussion or prolonged post-concussion symptoms acceptable? Are the potential long-term cognitive risks acceptable in exchange for future career (vocational, financial, and athletic) aspirations and goals? This approach, of course, takes the burden from the provider and puts it on the athlete and his or her parents.

In a comprehensive review of the long history of retirement-from-play recommendations in sports medicine, University of Colorado physiatrist Scott Laker and his co-authors offer a reasonable set of recommendations that stress the importance of neuropsychological testing and brain imaging for athletes being considered for retirement. They recommend retirement if neuropsychological testing shows persistent cognitive deficits, neurological examination shows abnormalities, or brain imaging shows brain hemorrhages or an Arnold Chiari malformation (a congenital abnormality of the cerebellum with protrusion into the opening in the skull—see Chapter 3).

The shared goals of providers, athletes, and parents are sometimes biased toward returning the athlete to play before the season ends. Therefore, the sports concussion clinic venue may not provide the most objective assessment for determining either return to play or retirement from a sport. The stakes—obtaining or keeping a college scholarship—are high for some players, such as Carla or Tom.

Prevention: The Name of the Game

The risk of repetitive or recurrent concussions for athletes remains an overriding worry: when someone sustains more than one concussion, their risk of long-term problems rises. We know that the younger the child or teenage athlete, the more likely they will experience recurrent concussions as they continue in their sport. Given the vulnerability of the immature brain, we make a major mistake when we put young people in harm's way by sending them back.

Can we significantly reduce the concussion risk in collision sports, especially for children and youth? Many sports organizations have adopted policies, guidelines, and rule changes on the field to decrease the risk of concussion, although the jury is still out as to what approaches bear the most fruit. Pop Warner, USA Football, the National Federation of State High School Associations (NFHS), and the National Collegiate Athletic Association (NCAA) update their policies, guidelines, and rules as researchers provide more evidence. But teams do not consistently comply with these protocols. Not surprisingly, given striking economic inequality in the United States, the affluent fare better than the poor. Equally unsurprising evidence shows that schools in poorer neighborhoods have fewer resources to implement concussion education and management strategies.

Medical organizations have not been willing to address key questions. For example, public health researcher Kathleen Bachynsky pointed out in a 2016 *New England Journal of Medicine* editorial that the AAP has not come out against youth tackle football despite evidence that eliminating tackling reduces concussions and catastrophic injuries. She reviewed the history of youth football in the 1950s, when the AAP recommended that children 12 years of age or younger not play body-contact sports, including tackle football, although at that time the recommendation's purpose was to reduce the risk of bone and joint injuries.

It may be possible to prevent some sports concussions with comprehensive pre-season physical examinations and carefully designed conditioning and strengthening programs to ensure that athletes' fitness can withstand the sports' demands on their bodies and reaction time. Pre-season physical exams should identify any history of prior injuries as well as medical conditions that might affect a player's athletic ability or present real dangers. Baseline cognitive testing enables comparison with a post-injury test should a concussion occur, although this is not always reliable. State laws regarding preparticipation physical examinations for student athletes vary. Coaches, athletic trainers, and physicians should ensure that athletes are physically prepared, and that athletic equipment is of high quality, meets standards, and is properly and individually fitted. Education about the rules of the sport and good sportsmanship must also form a key part of organized pre-season prevention activities.

The position the athlete plays, how aggressively they play, and their body positions, techniques, and equipment make certain players more vulnerable. Certain player positions may carry higher risks. In football, for example, there seems to be a higher than average concussion risk for collegiate linebackers, offensive linemen, and defensive backs. High school quarterbacks, linebackers, offensive linemen, tight ends, and defensive backs also have high risk. *Sports Illustrated* writer John Underwood, author of *Death of an American Game,* argued in the 1970s that football was too violent and overly commercialized. In 1976, the NFL, the NCAA, and the NFHS barred spearing (deliberately hitting another player with the crown of the helmet) or any head-down contact directed at another player. Players are not permitted to use the top of their helmets for blocking, hitting, tackling, or ball carrying.

Nevertheless, helmet-to-helmet contact is inevitable in tackle football, and strictly following and enforcing the rules has been a challenge for players. Research suggests that penalizing helmet-to-helmet contact, outlawing hits to a receiver, eliminating high-risk formations such as wedges during kickoffs, and limiting contact practices may reduce the frequency of football-related concussions. Limiting these contacts in youth football practices has demonstrated some promising results for reducing the frequency of head impacts, but there is no evidence that it reduces concussions. Unfortunately, at least so far, there is not convincing evidence that tackling technique training such as the USA Football "heads up" technique or rugby-style tackling leads to lower concussion rates in young athletes or in professional rugby players. On the other hand, Zachary Kerr, an epidemiologist at Indiana University, found evidence for better outcomes if a player safety coach was added to the program (to enforce proper blocking and tackling techniques).

Other rule changes might lower concussion rates. In a research letter to the *Journal of the American Medical Association*, Douglas Wiebe and fellow researchers noted that simple rule changes in Ivy League football—such as moving the kickoff position from the thirty-five-yard line to the forty-yard line and moving touchbacks from the twenty-five-yard line to the twenty-yard line—reduced concussions from eleven to two per thousand plays. Carolyn Emery at the University of Alberta and her research colleagues found that body checking in youth hockey led to a reduced risk of concussion in 11- and 12-year-olds.

Concussion rates in football are highest during games, but the actual number of concussions is higher for practices, because there are many more practices than games. The cumulative exposure to head impacts may lower the threshold for a concussion in football players, as Medical College of Wisconsin's Brian Stemper and his colleagues showed in a NCAA–Department of Defense study. In 2016, eight Ivy League schools voted to suspend tackling in football practice. Dartmouth set the example in 2010, bringing pads and tackling dummies, and even virtual players, onto the athletic field for practices. Their athletes experienced fewer concussions and still competed well. In soccer and basketball, sports where collisions are less integral to play, the numbers may be more equal. So, limiting contact in practice may be an effective strategy in only some sports.

University of Colorado epidemiologist Dawn Comstock and her staff analyzed data from the High School RIO (an internet-based data collection tool used in the National High School Sports-Related Injury Surveillance Study) to study high school sports-related injuries, with a goal of prevention. The researchers found that heading in soccer causes fewer concussions than player-to-player contact, especially among boys: two-thirds of soccer-related concussions in boys occur when players collide. Among girls, the number is half that. Substantially fewer concussions among high school boys (only about a third) involve heading, and even fewer involve heading for girls (one-quarter fewer). Perhaps calling fouls more frequently and changing other play rules would result in fewer concussions, although collision sports are just that—collision sports.

A class-action lawsuit filed in 2014 by parents and former players against the United States Soccer Federation was settled in 2015, and the organization banned players aged 10 and younger from heading the ball. The organization also restricted the number of headers in the 11 to 13 age group. A class action lawsuit against the NCAA aims to force similar changes in college soccer. Stricter enforcement of removal from the game ("red cards") for high elbows in heading duels in professional soccer is also associated with a reduced risk of concussion.

Sports-related concussions do not happen only during football or soccer practices and games, despite the fact that these sports receive the most research funding and media attention. The Institute of Medicine and National Research Council of the National Academies concluded that ice hockey, field hockey, wrestling, and lacrosse are at least as risky for athletes as football, and of course many young people participate in these sports. Although in general cheerleading carries an overall lower concussion risk than other sports, cheerleaders who perform stunts and pyramids carry the highest catastrophic injury risk of any young athletes. Bases have the highest rate of concussion in cheerleading, followed by flyers and spotters, with tumblers having the lowest rate.

Kelly Sarmiento, Dana Waltzman, and their CDC colleagues conducted two reviews of research studies on the prevention of sports concussion. One review focused on cultural aspects such as underreporting, lack of knowledge and education, and the attitudes of coaches and athletes toward concussion and concussion protocols. In one study, the CDC researchers found that most of the prevention research in six sports (football, ice hockey, soccer, lacrosse, basketball, and wrestling) focused on risk factors and secondary prevention, not the more important topic of primary prevention. They urged researchers to focus on primary prevention (focusing on reducing concussions) among young athletes. More work clearly needs to be done.

Legislation

Policy changes requiring legislation at state levels have addressed prevention. Concussion legislation began with the Zachery Lystedt Law passed in Washington State in 2009. Since then, all 50 states and the District of Columbia have enacted some form of concussion law, although these laws vary greatly, as does their implementation and enforcement. The Lystedt Law requires that school districts and athletic associations develop concussion guidelines and educational programs to increase awareness about the symptoms of concussion and disseminate "when in doubt, sit it out" messages. The law also mandates that youth athletes and a parent or guardian sign and return an information sheet annually, before the athlete's first practice or competition.

Unfortunately, state laws do not consistently include a mandate for educating coaches, athletic trainers, student athletes, and parents. Others do not even require that schools notify parents of a suspected concussion. Concussion laws that apply to public, private, and charter schools, sports organizations using public school property, or public recreational facilities vary from state to state. Although many laws are on the books, laws do not implement themselves, and even the strongest lack systems for monitoring and enforcement.

There is, however, some good news. Concussion reporting and diagnosis of concussions have surged, in part because of state legislation. Once state laws were enacted, the rate of concussion diagnosis went up. Carla and Tom were injured before concussion laws addressing removal and return to play were in place. Carla's incomplete recovery from her first concussion significantly contributed to the problems that ensued after her second soccer-related concussion. Tom had been hit on the field many times, beginning at age 12, before the concussion that forced his retirement from football.

Most state concussion laws require a written clearance from a licensed health-care provider who has the authority to clear an athlete to return to play. Some states require that a physician serve in this role, but other states grant this authority to a wide range of health-care providers: a registered nurse, athletic trainer, neuropsychologist, or physical therapist can play this role in some states. Access to providers trained in concussion management may be scarce, especially in rural areas. In 2017, North Carolina considered legislation that would permit parents to make the decision, although happily that proposal did not become law.

Equipment and Biomechanics

In the late nineteenth century, American football players wore padded leather helmets and shoulder pads under lightweight cotton jerseys and pants. Chin straps and face masks were added in the 1950s and 1960s, but despite the protective gear, football continued to have a reputation for catastrophic brain and spinal cord injuries and deaths. In the 1970s and 1980s, fatalities decreased when players began wearing improved and harder helmets that protected the bony structures of the head and neck and prevented the most severe brain injuries.

The research community agrees that while helmets prevent skull fractures, they do not eliminate the risk of brain injury from movement of the brain within the skull, rather than simple impact to the skull's exterior. That dichotomy—protection against fracture but not concussion—also holds for scrum hats, the headgear worn by rugby players. Badly fitting or wrongly sized headgear may, in fact, increase the risk of a concussion—the helmet can come off during an impact, or it can fail to protect vulnerable parts of a player's head. Helmets on young children may cause a "bobble-head" effect—nodding and shaking of the brain due to weaker neck muscles in relation to the size of the head and helmet.

Properly fitted sports equipment can prevent injuries. In a 2015 closed-door meeting, the National Operating Committee on Standards for Athletic Equipment (NOCSAE) acknowledged that for 95 percent of children, helmets are too heavy. NOCSAE receives much of its funding from sports equipment manufacturers. Standards for manufacturing and certifying football helmets have changed little over forty years. Two main manufacturers, Riddell and SG, compete in this marketplace. SG was acquired by the company LIGHT Helmets in 2019, a company that aims to make the lightest yet most protective helmet. There is definitely a market for better helmets and other sports equipment, but the risks of concussion will not be eliminated in collision sports.

Accelerometers and gyroscopes can be mounted on helmets and mouthguards to measure force, location, number, and direction during impacts. Sensors have been placed in clips, skin patches, skullcaps, and headbands as well as embedded in helmets or mouthpieces, and they can alert coaches and medical personnel about potentially dangerous hits. Collecting ongoing data about hits that may generate symptoms over time if not immediately can aid research. A force of 98 g is often the threshold for alerts, because concussions typically occur at 100 g. Multiple forces of 60 g, however, may eventually result in symptoms. While sensors measure impact to the helmet, jaw, or head, they may not correlate with impacts to the brain. Mechanisms in concussion include not just direct impacts from linear acceleration or pressure, but also rotational acceleration or strain that sensors might not effectively measure.

For more than forty years, the only safety standard helmets had to pass was a vertical drop test that measures linear forces. That has changed with more research. Virginia Tech researchers Steven Rowson, Ray Daniel, Stefan Duma, and their research colleagues used accelerometers and gyroscopes to develop a system of helmet ratings based on g-force research. Virginia Tech's Summation of Test for the Analysis of Risk (STAR) rating of 1 is associated with an impact of 150 g, whereas a 5 STAR rating is associated with 75 g.

Many colleges have begun to use sensors, but the NFL no longer uses them because in 2015 the NFL and its Player Association decided the evidence was not strong enough to support their use. In fact, University of Michigan researcher Kathryn O'Connor and her co-investigators published a review of the status of these devices in 2017 and concluded that "head-impact-monitoring systems have limited clinical utility due to error rates, designs, and low specificity in predicting concussive injury." On the other hand, biomechanical research using sensor technology will continue to shed light on the science of concussion.

Actually, maybe using less sports equipment can make sports safer. Eric Swartz of the University of New Hampshire is leading a study of helmetless football. Preliminary results suggest that with proper training, education, and instruction, helmetless collegiate football players can safely perform supervised tackling and blocking drills during practice without helmets. Tackling without helmets may reduce the false sense of security a helmet provides. Not wearing a helmet may make athletes more cautious and less aggressive toward other players. Zachary Kerr and his fellow researchers in Indiana found that concussion practice rates for football were highest when the athletes were fully padded.

Turf, Temperature, and Altitude

External factors are always at play during athletic practice and games. Athletes are about as likely to hit the ground as they are to collide with another player, and often both occur in sequence. Therefore, another prevention measure relates to turf. Researchers studying sports injuries rate a playing field's shock absorbency with a metric called Gmax. An object that approximates a human head and neck (about twenty square inches and twenty pounds) dropped from a height of two feet for a Gmax score of 1 forms the basis for turf testing methods.

Grass has a Gmax score of just over 60. Playing fields are supposed to have a Gmax score of 200 or less, according to ASTM International (formerly known as the American Society for Testing and Materials, a technical standards organization). Gmax testing measures the shock-attenuation performance of sports turf, both artificial and natural. Gmax performance is measured as the ratio of the maximum acceleration / deceleration rate relative to the rate of acceleration due to the earth's gravity. Athletic turf should be tested annually because surfaces change over time. Construction materials and methods, maintenance, weather, soil, other environmental conditions, and frequency and type of use can all affect the resulting Gmax score.

Toronto researcher David Lawrence and his colleagues found that colder temperatures may heighten the risk of sports concussion (and ankle injuries) in the NFL. A number of researchers have been investigating whether altitude may affect concussion rates, perhaps by increasing cerebral blood flow to the brain. For example, Gregory Myer at Cincinnati Children's Hospital and his research group reported that data from the NFL and high school teams (football, baseball, wrestling, volleyball, soccer, and basketball) support this theory. He is researching the Q-collar, a device worn around the neck that compresses the internal jugular vein to increase blood flow to the head and decrease "sloshing" (movement of the brain within the skull). Physiologists James Smoliga and Gerald Zavorsky want to put this research to rest. They argue that the studies are flawed and that even at very high altitudes (13,000 feet), brains don't change in ways that would support the research. And the mile-high stadium in Denver, Colorado, they argue, should have no effect on a football player's brain.

What Now?

When Carla and Tom professed their love of sport, they never mentioned money or politics. They talked about the sheer joy of teamwork and physical and mental exertion for a common goal, underscoring the benefits of striving to perform at their personal best by summoning the physical and mental energy at practice, again and again—a process of honing skills and focus that can lead to exhilarating success. Their parents wanted them to participate for "character building"—to develop resiliency, self-discipline, and the grit to get up and try again after being knocked down. These young athletes found the virtue of sport obvious. For example, conversations with her mother had taught Carla that Title IX provided her with opportunities that her mother, a field-hockey goalie, never dreamed of. Tom had a hunch that corporations he might want to work for would rate his football past as a factor as important as his grade point average. Carla and Tom also avidly followed their sports as spectators and deeply admired the individual professional athletes who served as their role models.

Many Americans gather to cheer on their high school football teams on Friday nights—there are towns in Texas where local football verges on a religion, and there are towns in Indiana where the same is true for basketball. In small communities, friendships and business alliances form around what serves, despite intense rivalries, as a relatively nonpolarizing activity, enabling neighbors to socialize comfortably, especially when other issues such as politics and culture have become more and more partisan. Tailgating parties and sports bars can even bring the fans of opposing teams together, at least some of the time.

Sports spectator fervor cements our collective admiration for the finest athletes, past and present, who represent the physical, mental, and moral capacities we all aspire to—agility, endurance, fortitude, focus, commitment, perseverance, loyalty, camaraderie, and community. We place high expectations on athletes as modern heroes. Role models in other sectors of public and political life often fall short of our ideals. When sports heroes falter, fall, or fail to represent the best capacities of human beings, we may forgive them more easily—even gods can turn out to have clay feet. Nelson Mandela, former president of South Africa and co-winner (with F. W. de Klerk) of the Nobel Peace Prize in 1993, said this about sports: "Sports have the power to change the world. It has the power to inspire, the power to unite people in a way that little else does. It speaks to youth in a language they understand. Sports can create hope, where there was once only despair. It is more powerful than governments in breaking down racial barriers. It laughs in the face of all types of discrimination."

After extolling the virtues of sports, however, we must face the fact that there are injuries resulting from sports. Concussions represent a public health concern, especially repeat concussions. The health risks associated with collision sports for players subjected to multiple hits are quite high. Young athletes playing a collision sport may incur hundreds and thousands of hits without an actual concussion diagnosis. I can't stress enough that a previous concussion can significantly increase the risk of another, and then another. Although interventions to lower risk may help, nothing can lower the risk to zero in collision sports other than eliminating collisions and thus changing the nature of the sport. We must protect our young people, and this may require difficult decisions about what sports they play and at what age they play them.

Time-Out and Time's Up

Sports culture is undergoing change, and more of us now have a greater awareness of concussion's potential for short- and long-term consequences. There are signs that people are paying attention. Parents are worrying more about the risks of collision sports and have begun making decisions for their children on that basis. Some schools have eliminated football due to decreased enthusiasm for the sport or parental worry. However, other collision sports with concussion risks—soccer, hockey, and lacrosse—and high-risk sports such as wrestling, gymnastics, and cheerleading, have not seen declines in participation.

As with any public health concern, reducing risks of concussion depends upon education, advocacy, and legislation, as well as the ability and willingness of health-care professionals on the front lines, on the sidelines, on guideline committees, and in clinics to advise young people and their families about what we know and what is prudent, based on scientific evidence. Greater numbers of athletes are being removed from play when they experience a concussion or are observed having one, and the Lystedt Law and CDC resources have helped raise awareness.

A few experts have put their necks out to say no to certain athletic activities for young people. Neurosurgeon Robert Cantu believes tackle football, heading the ball in soccer, and full-body-checking in hockey are not safe for kids under 14. Pathologist Bennet Omalu suggests that we legislate a legal age of eighteen for contact sports in a *New York Times* editorial in 2015: "We have a legal age for drinking alcohol; for joining the military; for voting; for smoking; for driving; and for consenting to have sex. We must have the same when it comes to protecting the organ that defines who we are as human beings." Now we have even more evidence suggesting that the developing brain may not fully mature until we reach our late twenties. This might have to change our recommendations about contact and collision sports.

My own children are no longer at risk from youth sports, but my young grandchildren will be. In one way or another, we are all exposed to this public health crisis. After centuries of debate, decades of clinical guideline and consensus statements, and the passage of various state laws, we still lack a comprehensive national plan for the protection of young athletes. We need measures of the effectiveness of concussion legislation and education, and most important, systems of accountability and enforcement. It's definitely time for more teamwork to protect our young athletes.

7

Money Talks

ACCORDING TO A 2017 Gallup Poll, football has been America's favorite spectator sport since 1972, despite recent slippage. Today 37 percent of Americans rate football tops among all sports, down from a peak of over 40 percent in 2006 and 2007. By comparison, basketball earns 11 percent of viewers and baseball just 9 percent. The Gallup analysts proposed three probable reasons for football's decline in popularity since its peak. First, the National Football League (NFL) has been castigated for insufficiently disciplining players who assault their intimate partners, which came to light through a video released of running back Ray Rice's assault on his then fiancée. Second, some players created controversy by taking a knee during the national anthem. Third, the movie *Concussion* publicized the NFL's cover-up of the serious outcomes of players' head injuries (see Chapter 4). Despite these setbacks, 42 percent of men and 32 percent of women still say football is their favorite sport.

Wide Receiving

It's impossible to discuss sports in American society without considering the role of television. The first televised football game aired in 1938, and college football began broadcasting in 1939. The first dedicated sports channel aired in 1977, and the National Collegiate Athletic Association (NCAA) controlled television rights for college sporting events until 1984. ESPN began broadcasting two years later. Today, TV sports are local, national, and international, and everyone gets to choose their favorites on cable stations or streaming media. TV broadcasts provide lucrative revenues for college and university teams as well as for professional sports. For years, Sunday Night Football on NBC has been the top-rated show on any channel, and ESPN's Monday Night Football has been the number one cable show.

Combined US sports earnings measure in the tens of billions of dollars. Projections have the North American sports market growing at a compound annual rate of more than 3 percent from 2017 to 2021 across various economic segments—media rights, gate revenues, sponsorship, and merchandizing—until it reaches $78.5 billion by 2022. The US sports industry as a whole is growing much faster than the national gross domestic product (GDP).

American football reaps the highest profits of any sport. The NFL operates as a monopoly exempt from antitrust legislation and brings in more than $10 billion a year. In 1961, President John F. Kennedy signed legislation to allow professional football teams to jointly negotiate radio and television broadcast rights. In 1966, Congress approved the merger of the NFL with the American Football

League, extending the antitrust exemption. That year, CBS paid $2 million to broadcast the championship game.

The Internal Revenue Service gave the NFL a financial boost in 1961 when it expanded its definition of nonprofit entities to include professional sports leagues. NFL headquarters paid no taxes in New York until 2015, when the NFL finally lost its tax-exempt status. Over decades, the NFL and other sports leagues have benefited from millions in taxpayer subsidies to build stadiums. Fans also pay for their favorite sports teams through cable subscriptions that automatically include sports channels in most basic packages. These phenomena essentially tax people who do not watch sports to subsidize those who do.

Spectator sports appear to be recession-proof. Like alcohol sales, sports revenues continued to soar during the Great Recession. NFL Commissioner Roger Goodell pledged to his thirty-two team owners that the league would grow to $25 billion in revenue by 2027, increasing $1 billion each year starting in 2016. Perhaps people need sports more than ever as an antidote to depressing economic and political news, and maybe sports compensate for other deprivations. Whatever the reason, most other entertainment industries do not come close to producing $75 billion in revenue, with only one competitor reaping more—$100 billion from video gaming. Fantasy sports also generate major revenue, with about 60 million participants.

Although scandals and other issues have trimmed his salary, Commissioner Goodell still earned over $30 million in 2015, the year the NFL voluntarily relinquished its tax-exempt status largely because of political pressure. The contract Goodell negotiated in 2018 will yield him $200 million over five years. Indeed, in a contest of CEOs, Goodell wins the game by turning a $900 million business in 2006 into a multi-billion-dollar business in 2019. According to *Forbes,* only ten S&P CEOs made more than $40 million in 2016, and Goodell has joined this group.

Big Money on Campus

The seduction of sports money also exists on college campuses. College sports fuel the pipeline to professional sports. There are now five immensely influential college sports conferences, dubbed the Power Five: the Atlantic Coast Conference (ACC), Big Ten Conference (BIG), Big 12 Conference, Pac-12 Conference, and Southeastern Conference (SEC). Most Big Ten institutions are large state universities with enrollments of 30,000 or more students, and all have financial endowments. Big Ten schools educate more than half a million students each year and count approximately 6 million living alumni.

The Power Five conferences' wealthiest athletic departments pulled in a record $6 billion in 2017, nearly $4 billion more than all other schools combined. These schools procure multi-million-dollar media rights and fill their coffers with ticket-sales revenues. As an example, the University of Texas Longhorns receive Big 12 money, boast a 100,000-seat football stadium, and hold a twenty-year, $300 million ESPN contract. Texas A&M tops Texas's college sports annual revenue at more than $190 million, and the University of Texas ranks a close second.

Not surprisingly, football generates most of the revenue in Texas college sports. Public universities such as Alabama, Florida, Louisiana State University, Michigan, Ohio State, Oklahoma, Penn State, Tennessee, and Wisconsin, and private schools like Notre Dame and the University of Southern California (USC), also bring in enormous revenues for their campuses. Eight of these schools have stadiums that seat at or close to one hundred thousand, with Michigan's Big House official capacity of 107,601 the largest. As a friend who teaches at Michigan said to me as we drove by the stadium, "Football is the religion here, and that is our cathedral." College football teams in states that lack professional teams, like Nebraska, Oklahoma, and South Carolina, pick up the slack to fill stadiums with avid fans. Wealthy schools spend money on private jets and five-star hotels, whether to recruit athletes or for team or executive use, and some athletic department staff take home seven-figure salaries, far more than the faculty members earn at these same institutions.

Power Five and Group of Five schools have seen substantial increases in net revenues for years. The smaller conference schools that make up the Group of Five have moved hundreds of millions of dollars from taxpayers, students, and other university programs into their athletic programs. About half the revenue for public school athletic departments in the Group of Five comes from student fees, university subsidies, and state or local governments. And like the Super Bowl, college bowl games garner vast audiences and result in huge television revenues.

Big Little Leagues

Youth sports have always had a place in the money-sports-politics nexus, which has been termed the sports-industrial complex. Title IX, a 1972 federal law which stipulates that no person be excluded on the basis of sex from programs receiving federal funds, has had the effect of increasing participation and support for public and private high school sports programs. Whereas Pop Warner and Little League Baseball memberships have dropped, private sports club memberships are climbing. Across the country, parents sign up children as young as 4 for sports camps and athletic events, and invest in coaching, travel opportunities, and equipment to increase their skill level. According to WinterGreen Research, youth sports is a $17 billion market in the United States, about the same amount as the NFL's. *Time* reports that small towns and municipalities count on private youth sports complexes to boost their economies. Winter-Green Research projects that these markets will reach $57.8 billion by 2024.

Although only 2 percent of high school athletes play at the top college level, some parents feel that an investment before high school may be worth the high price tag. These parents may part with the equivalent of a year of college tuition for their 8- or 9-year-old to prepare for the day that high school and college scouts show up to observe young talent. Joel Brenner and the American Academy of Pediatrics cautions against pre-adolescent sports specialization, stating that burnout, anxiety, depression and attrition are increased in early specializers, but that has not deterred eager parents and kids.

The Players' Stakes

Any discussion of money in the sports-industrial complex must include the money players make, may make, or risk losing. Many college athletes receive significant financial benefits, such as tuition reimbursement, room and board, and other perks in exchange for helping to bring in huge revenues for colleges. Debates rage in the media, among legislators, and in the courts regarding whether, how, and how much college players should be compensated on campuses. Decisions about payment for allegedly "amateur" college players bring to bear union organizing, right-to-work state legislation, NCAA rules, and other factors for both public and private schools, adding yet another layer of financial complexity to the love, money, and politics equation.

There are always incentives to play and keep playing. For high schoolers, the carrot is a college scholarship and its attendant perks. For the high-performing college athlete, it's a chance at the pros.

What could that financial reward potentially be? The average NFL player makes about 2 million dollars per year, and football players' active careers are shorter than those of professional athletes in other sports. The average for other national professional sports associations is much higher, ranging from about 3 million to 6 million. Few incentives, other than the prospect of good health into old age, exist for any competitive athlete at the high school, college, or professional level to report symptoms of concussion or other injuries if they are mild enough to hide. A majority of players in any sport, especially those we rarely hear or read about at the college or professional level, make little money over their sports careers. But they stand to lose their shot at a big paycheck if they can't stay in a game or play during the next game or the one after that. Any negative label suggesting weakness or injury risks their careers.

Moving to Center Field

With so much at stake financially, and so much to lose, the NFL and other sports organizations have been less than forthcoming about the long-lasting effects of injury. For many years, the NFL and its physician leaders have deflected claims about the dangers of concussion on the football field. In 1994, then NFL commissioner Paul Tagliabue, who called concussions "a journalism issue" (although he later apologized), created the NFL Mild Traumatic Brain Injury Committee, appointing his personal physician, Elliot Pellman, a rheumatologist, to head it. Although his specialty did not include the study of traumatic brain injury (TBI), Pellman also served as a physician for the New York Jets, so he was acquainted with concussion. The NFL Mild Traumatic Brain Injury Committee and Pellman co-authored a series of fifteen articles, as well as guidelines, on concussion published in *Neurosurgery* between 2003 and 2009.

Using NFL data, they argued that concussions carry no risk and have no long-term consequences.

In 2005, Bennet Omalu published the results of Pittsburgh Steelers center Mike Webster's autopsy, and the Mild Traumatic Brain Injury Committee opined that returning an athlete to play after a concussion did not involve significant risks of another injury either in the same game or during the season. For years, *Neurosurgery* and other journals and medical and sports organizations continued to promote the belief that concussions are transient and that brain structures remain intact after blows to the head. *Neurosurgery* researchers received funding from the NFL and other sports organizations, and initially no one paid particular attention to the conflicts of interest (COIs) inherent in this marriage of sports, medicine, and science.

Researchers without ties to the NFL later called the researchers' COIs into question and discredited their conclusions. In 1999, before his death in 2002, the NFL retirement board finally acknowledged Webster's claim that the concussions he suffered while playing produced his later dementia. But during the 1990s, when Webster struggled to subsist, declining in mental and physical health, the NFL Mild Traumatic Brain Injury Committee chaired by Pellman deliberated over whether concussions were serious, and if and when concussed athletes should be removed from play or evaluated by a medical professional.

A turning point occurred for NFL players when, in their class action lawsuit against the NFL, 5,000 plaintiffs, all former players, argued that the NFL knew about CTE risks from repetitive concussions yet covered up research findings. In 2011 court documents, the NFL admitted that it expected 28 percent of retired players, nearly one in three, to develop a neurodegenerative disease. The NFL anticipated that more than 6,000 of its retirees will be diagnosed with one of the health conditions identified in the settlement: Alzheimer's disease and other forms of dementia, Parkinson's, and amyotrophic lateral sclerosis (ALS, or Lou Gehrig's disease).

The NFL also agreed that players are likely to be diagnosed at younger ages than individuals in the general population with the same conditions. While the absolute numbers are small, the differences loom large. For example, players younger than 50 have a 0.8 percent chance of developing dementia, compared with a less than 0.1 percent chance for the general population. Players in the age group 50 to 54 have an estimated rate of 1.4 percent, compared with less than 0.1 percent for the general population. Further, players with milder cognitive problems are unlikely to receive any money from the settlement unless their condition deteriorates to dementia.

As part of the agreement, the NFL will pay out $1 billion (or possibly more) over sixty-five years. While this seems a staggering amount of money, this settlement represents a mere fraction of NFL revenue. And the NFL players' settlement covers only players who retired by January 7, 2014. Approximately 22,000 retired players had to undergo baseline testing before August 2017. Only the families of players who have died, and only if they received a postmortem examination that diagnosed CTE, may receive a payout. Mike Webster's family may not get a cent because he died before the settlement was reached.

In December 2016, the Supreme Court declined to hear appeals filed over these exclusions, so the lower court decision stands. However, Senior US District Court Judge Anita Brody ordered the parties to revisit the settlement as the science of CTE advances. Some ex-players opted out and plan instead to pursue individual lawsuits. The settlement committee mandated creation of a list of physicians qualified to conduct evaluations, and the court directed that no NFL-affiliated physicians may be included on this list, a recognition by the court of the COI problem that has plagued sports concussion research and practice. The NFL case remains complicated, with court decisions making the news as claims are filed, denied, appealed, and audited.

In March 2016, Jeff Miller, NFL senior vice president for health and safety, testified before the US House of Representatives' Committee on Energy and Commerce about football player health and safety. Representative Jan Schakowsky asked Miller if the link between football and neurodegenerative diseases such as CTE has been established, and Miller said "certainly yes," adding that more research is needed. This was the NFL's first official admission of the major problem the sport faces.

The NCAA, the organization that includes over 1,100 colleges and universities with varsity sports programs, has also faced concussion litigation. In 2014, the NCAA reached a proposed settlement that included $70 million for testing former athletes over the next fifty years to monitor the long-term consequences of concussion, and an additional $5 million for concussion-related research. The settlement requires schools to make changes to their concussion protocols and return-to-play policies. Unlike the NFL settlement, the NCAA decision doesn't include medical cost compensation for former athletes. A month after that settlement was reached, San Diego State University football player Anthony Nichols challenged it for not directly compensating athletes. Another settlement permits former athletes to sue their colleges and universities, conferences, and the NCAA for financial compensation.

The count of individual lawsuits continues to grow as more and more athletes suffer concussions and their long-term consequences.

The Health-Care Industrial Complex

Less noticeable than the sports-industrial complex is a similar nexus of money and influence which we might term the health-care industrial complex. This complex also holds stakes in what happens when we discuss concussion. The National Operating Committee on Standards for Athletic Equipment (NOCSAE) is one example. The committee was founded in 1969 largely with funding from helmet manufacturers "to commission research directed toward injury reduction in sports." Importantly, the NOCSAE does not certify equipment; rather, it funds research and sets standards. Since 1978, NCAA rules mandate the use of certified helmets, and the National Federation of State High School Associations has required the use of helmets certified to the NOCSAE standards for high school play since 1980.

Researchers and others argue that youth helmets are too big and too heavy, and some have criticized NOCSAE for delaying safety standards for youth helmets and other equipment. Some have also criticized the organization's failure to counter the helmet-industry argument that third-party aftermarket accessories, such as impact sensors or additional padding, raise certification and liability concerns for football's governing bodies. Researchers have also faulted NOCSAE for funding the research of its board members without requiring a peer-review process.

Individuals as well as organizations such as these may have significant COIs. These people may include sports medicine doctors, other physicians and other health-care personnel and researchers who serve on sports organization boards and governing bodies, safety committees for equipment companies (such as helmet and impact sensor manufacturers), boards of corporations that sponsor or run ads on sports broadcasts, and clinical practice guideline committees. Some of these individuals have benefited financially from developing, using, and promoting computerized testing materials and from media exposure, including television shows, film documentaries, and book sales, or from speaking at congressional hearings and testifying in court. Remuneration for these activities may take the form of salaries, consultation or legal fees, or simply reimbursement for expenses. The total price tag for physicians and other clinicians who participate directly in the business of sport through team or league employment and other sports-related businesses remains unknown, but we can surmise that it is high.

In 2014, the American Academy of Neurology (AAN) published a position paper written by neurologist Matthew Kirschen and a team of researchers. The authors discuss the legal and ethical considerations of sports-related concussion, and argue that "Ideally, physician reimbursement pertaining to sports-related concussion should be solely derived from patient evaluation, management, and counseling activities," and, in addition, "they and other members of concussion management teams (e.g., physical therapists and neuropsychologists) should disclose all financial arrangements that could influence patient care decisions to athletes and parents, including contractual relationships with teams, organizations, or governing bodies, involvement (scientific or financial) in the development of diagnostic or protective equipment, or paid sponsorships." The paper emphasizes the physician's primary responsibility: "to protect the health and well-being of their patients, regardless of financial interests or employment considerations."

The NFL pays medical professionals to care for its players on and off the field. The physicians and athletic trainers employed by the league make key decisions about removal from play or return to play. With funding from the NFL players' union and as part of the Football Players Health Study at Harvard, a group of lawyers published a report in 2016, "Protecting and Promoting the Health of NFL Players: Legal and Ethical Analysis and Recommendations," that addresses potential issues surrounding COIs for doctors on team payrolls. The report argues that physicians who work for professional football teams have COIs that could put the teams' business interests ahead of players' health.

This report identifies seventy-six recommendations aimed at twenty stakeholders. The primary recommendation is that there be "division of responsibilities" between a player's physician and the club's physician, suggesting that a joint committee with representatives from both the NFL and NFL Players Association appoint players' physicians, and club physicians be permitted to evaluate players only for business purposes (for example, deciding whether to offer a player a contract). In response, the NFL argued that this recommendation is "untenable" and "impractical" and that it would have "unintended but extremely detrimental effects on NFL players' care."

The Harvard study group did not stop with this publication. Two other reports, "A Proposal to Address NFL Club Doctors' Conflicts of Interest and Promote Player Trust" (a Hastings Center publication) and "Evaluating NFL Player Health and Performance: Legal and Ethical Issues," add to a growing literature that addresses not only NFL players' health but the health of other athletes. Although they find fault with procedures within the NFL, the authors also credit the NFL for doing more than other sports leagues to protect their athletes.

The Case of Guidelines

Over the last forty years, many organizations in the United States and abroad have written guidelines for sports-related concussions that provide scientific reviews, practice recommendations, and reassurance to clinicians that their decisions are consistent with those of others. Medical societies or their representatives usually convene guideline panels, and concussion guidelines are ultimately created primarily through consensus. Often, not enough research exists to codify diagnosis, treatment, and prognostication.

Concussion guideline experts have for the most part been physicians—orthopedists, sports medicine specialists, neurologists, neurosurgeons, and physiatrists. Many hold strong beliefs that the benefits of sports activities for young people outweigh the risks. The groups that produce these documents usually lack diverse or dissenting views. Some members have major COIs, and some groups include only one pathologist weighing in about CTE, for example. It should come as no surprise that sports medicine physicians and others who serve on these research and guideline committees tend to enjoy playing and watching sports. In the case of concussion guidelines, they may be serving their own interests by reassuring players and their families that school-based sports are safe.

When organizations recruit panelists or reviewers for developing guidelines, they require disclosure of potential or real COIs. As more and more research money flows from sports leagues and equipment manufacturers to organizations, researchers, and clinicians who develop guidelines, it is difficult to find experts who do not have potential or real COIs. Attention falls largely on direct payments, but clinician and researcher activities also usually garner indirect compensation, such as travel or other expense reimbursement for meetings. COIs have an enormous potential to bias sports research and clinical guidelines.

To be fair, many people have difficulty recognizing their own biases, so disclosure of a potential conflict at least reveals the existence of possible contributions to bias. The Harvard researchers who published *Protecting and Promoting the Health of NFL Players* note that individuals and organizations may identify potential COIs and design a structure of rules, procedures, incentives, and controls to minimize them. A "consider the opposite" strategy, others suggest, is one way to turn the tables on personal interests or beliefs by forcing individuals to argue an opposing view. Perhaps guideline committees should also deliberately choose people who actually hold opposing and diverse points of view.

The biggest question of all may be this: how can a COI be resolved? Is it sufficient simply to disclose its existence, as is typically the case for professional medical activities such as speaking engagements or membership on boards? Some ethicists argue that the bias caused by such COIs, and the near-impossibility of maintaining objectivity in the face of that bias, is a key concern. But what constitutes a bias? If a physician-researcher is an avid football fan, or a coach or former professional player volunteers in their community's after-school sports program, does their enthusiasm or experience in itself make them unable to interpret research findings clearly or be objective when serving on an expert panel to create a clinical guideline?

The history of concussion guidelines underscores that using consensus-only criteria may be harmful and limiting, even if the organizations and members of guideline panels are well-intentioned and thorough in examining evidence. Guidelines based on consensus have been used over many decades for deciding whether an athlete can continue to play now or in the future, and these decisions have affected thousands of athletes. Guidelines help raise awareness about concussion and its risks, but they should be developed by those who have no vested interest in the sport.

The earliest guidelines relied on ill-defined terms such as "mild," "moderate," and "severe"—unquantifiable terms open to competing interpretations. Boston neurosurgeon Robert Cantu, a longtime physician to athletes with concussions, was the primary author of the 1986 concussion guidelines published in *Neurosurgery*. In 1997, an American Academy of Neurology (AAN) expert panel created another set of guidelines with another grading system, based primarily on loss of consciousness and length of resolution of signs and symptoms. No research backed up the grading system or the notion that loss of consciousness itself means a more severe injury occurred. Newer guidelines and consensus statements abandon grading systems altogether. Instead, they recommend adopting an "individualized approach" to concussion diagnosis and treatment.

Guideline authors have also been reticent to acknowledge the young brain's vulnerability to long-term and sometimes permanent consequences from sports concussion. With funding from sports organizations, including the Fédération Internationale de Football Association (FIFA) and the International Olympics Committee (IOC), a group of experts with an extensive list of COI disclosures met at the 5th International Conference on Concussion in Berlin in October 2016. In April 2017, they published a consensus statement in the *British Medical Journal* that skirts the question of long-term concussion consequences, including the big one: CTE. The statement concludes: "There is much more to learn about the potential cause-and-effect relationships of repetitive head impact exposure, concussions, and long-term brain health." This oft-repeated statement comes to mind: "Absence of evidence is not evidence of absence."

Guidelines also avoid other key questions. What credentials, expertise, and training should the person have who decides when and for how long to sideline a player during practice or games? How extensive should initial testing or examinations be for an athlete with a concussion? What physicians, and from what specialties, and what other licensed healthcare professionals, should have final authority to diagnose and decide about return to play and treatment?

Every US state and the District of Columbia now has laws regarding concussion, but there is no agreement about who should perform sideline assessments or who should diagnose and treat athletes or make return-to-play and retire-from-play decisions.

Position statements on physician COIs and professional ethics have not made headlines, but they may represent a trend. In 2016, the editorial board of the *Journal of Clinical Orthopedics and Related Research* took the striking position that orthopedic surgeons should recommend that children and young adults not play tackle football. Their 2017 editorial, "Do Orthopaedic Surgeons Belong on the Sidelines of American Football Games," concludes that "While concussions are not the area of first expertise of most orthopaedic surgeons, our presence on the sidelines helps this sport to continue. In light of the known risks, we suggest that surgeons evaluate whether continuing to support this sport is consonant with the best values of our profession. We believe it is not." It is unlikely that this recommendation reached a wide audience, even in the medical world. However, the statement makes a definite break from concussion guideline recommendations by physicians who suggest that football and other collision sports can continue for children and young adults without a significant threat to their health or welfare.

The End Games

As one outgrowth of concussion controversies and the legal quagmire it has spawned, the NFL, the NCAA, and other sports organizations have tried to make football safer. In 2009, the NFL banned same-game return to play after a concussion. Since then, changes in return-to-play protocols have evolved. The NFL put in place a league-wide protocol in 2011. A year later, league-placed spotters were tasked with identifying players with suspected concussions. By

2013, the NFL required independent neurologist evaluations before players could return to the field after a concussion. In 2016, the NFL and its players association announced their intent to enforce a protocol with fines and other disciplinary action for player violations.

Nevertheless, notably, Ken Belson reported in the *New York Times* in 2018 that the NFL also gave $45 million to USA Football in 2014 "to spread the gospel of football to jittery moms and dads." And Belson quoted David Baker, president of the Pro Football Hall of Fame: "If we lose football, we lose a lot in America. I don't know if America can survive." In other words, Baker claimed, football is inextricably tied to the future of America. In the end, protocols and player safety intertwine with the sports-industrial complex's goal of keeping football America's favorite sport.

Public health advocates Kathleen Bachynski and Daniel Goldberg point out that the CDC and the National Institutes of Health both have foundations that permit the receipt of millions of dollars of corporate money for research and educational programs and materials. This raises the possibility that sports organizations may exert undue influence on medical research. In fact, overt attempts to influence and even to distort research findings have occurred. Bachynski and Goldberg mention two notable examples. The first involves concussion education, a worthy endeavor. The NFL and USA Football's Heads Up Football educational program, initiated in 2003 in conjunction with the CDC, has provided a multitude of educational materials geared for students, parents, coaches, trainers, and school officials, and also operates a certification system for coaches. But when the organizations touted claims that the program dramatically reduced the rate of concussions, *New York Times* reporter Alan Schwarz strongly disagreed—the researchers and organizations then dropped the claim. Unfortunately, state, county, and school system rules vary, with few mandates for education, training, or certification, and it is not clear what effects these "optional" educational programs have had.

A second case involves research. The NFL has been one of the largest funders of brain research, a fact that has led to comparisons with the tobacco industry. Indeed, a substantial amount of this funding has gone to scientists and institutions affiliated with the NFL. In 2012, the NFL pledged a $30 million unrestricted gift to the National Institutes of Health. However, in 2016, the NFL withheld the funds for a $16 million study of CTE. Following reports that the NFL was backing out of its promises to make objective funding decisions, Democratic members of the House Committee on Energy and Commerce led an investigation. In the end, the Committee members argued that the NFL had attempted to steer the funding to a physician with ties to the NFL in order to influence the research. The NFL issued a statement rejecting the allegations and said the organization "is deeply committed to continuing to accelerate scientific research and advancements in this critical area, and we stand ready to support additional independent research to that end."

What Now?

The concussion spotlight has widened to encompass collision sports such as hockey, soccer, rugby, lacrosse, basketball, cheerleading, and others. Actually, cheerleaders rack up a high number of catastrophic injuries, similar to football. Even sports less associated with concussions such as wrestling, gymnastics, baseball, and softball belong on the list to watch. Watching the Olympics and Paralympics reminds us that concussion occurs with extreme sports as well. Winter sports such as downhill skiing, snowboarding, and figure skating and aquatic sports such as water skiing and water polo carry high risks, even for the fittest athletes. Organizations that govern these sports have been slower than the NFL to use standardized protocols and other interventions to identify, diagnose, and prevent concussions. Nor have they addressed and managed COIs. We clearly need more action from all the responsible leadership groups, including professional organizations, schools, and colleges, as well as from legislatures.

The Union of Concerned Scientists (UCS) produced a "Disinformation Playbook" that names five tactics used by businesses and business interests to "deceive, misinform, and buy influence at the expense of public health and safety." The UCS minces no words. We must carefully watch the entire sports industrial and health-care industrial complexes, and the public must awaken to the threats to science posed when sports, money, and politics play in the same arena. The UCS Playbook calls out counterfeit science (The Fake), harassment of scientists (The Blitz), manufacturing uncertainty (The Diversion), buying credibility through alliances with academia or professional societies (The Screen), and manipulation of government officials and bureaucratic processes (The Fix).

George Lundberg, the longtime editor of the *Journal of the American Medical Association* (*JAMA*), wrote an editorial, "Boxing Should be Banned in Civilized Countries," published on January 14, 1983. The editorial played an important role in changing the views of physicians, lawmakers, and eventually the public. On February 4, 2016, Lundberg explained his updated views in a *New York Times* commentary: "If the NFL can't effectively deal with the concussion issue, it may follow the same arc as boxing. That would be a shame. I have had a love affair with American football, especially Alabama football, since 1944, the legendary Harry Gilmer's first year. The only thing I love more than football is the human brain. Blows to the head damage the brain, period. It need not be a full concussion. We learned from decades of studying boxing that multiple subconcussive blows result in aggregate widespread tearing of nerve fibers and small blood vessels, and possibly to chronic traumatic encephalopathy."

Ray Fair at Yale and his co-author Christopher Champa calculated the cost savings if twelve college sports and five high school contact sports were changed to noncontact sports. The concussion numbers would drop by 6,900 per year for college athletes and 161,400 for high school athletes. They estimated the total injury savings in 2015 dollars as between $433 million and $1.5 million for college sports and between $5.1 and $18.4 million for high school sports. Expanding this to include women's sports would further advance the financial argument. That's not the only argument, of course, given the effect of injury on the lives of these student athletes and their families, but these injuries do have a price tag.

Polls suggest that while many parents have decided they don't want their sons playing football, most expect the game's popularity to continue unabated, and many continue to stream and watch football and other collision sports. In 2018, more than 75 percent of Super Bowl viewers surveyed by Burson-Marsteller (now Burson Cohn and Wolfe) said stories of concussions don't affect their viewing of the game, and they believe the NFL is making the sport safer.

Will the medical profession, the research community, public health officials, and sports organizations do the right thing and educate the public about the science of concussion? And will these groups have the courage to take an unbiased stand? Can private and public funders ramp up research and disseminate results in clearly understandable ways, so all of us can make informed decisions about sports participation? Serious questions about the health and welfare of all athletes, but especially young ones, beg for answers. For some questions, however, the information is already available, if we pay attention.

Part Three

Dangers at Home and Work

It is the business of the future to be dangerous; and it is among the merits of science that it equips its future for its duties.

—ALFRED NORTH WHITEHEAD, 1925

8

Close to Home

Concussion is a risk across the entire life span. Several patients come to mind and make the case for concussion being an equal-opportunity event. For example, Kali, age 2, was thriving and meeting all her milestones. Then, one late afternoon while her mother, Stephanie, prepared dinner, Kali wriggled out of the high chair and fell forward. Stephanie turned to find her thrashing around on the kitchen floor, screaming at the top of her lungs. Panicking, the young mother quickly grabbed her cell phone and called 911. Forty-five minutes later, Stephanie and Kali arrived at their local hospital.

Seventy-two-year-old Barbara taught college math for more than forty years before she retired at age 66. She was in good health except for atrial fibrillation, and she took warfarin daily to prevent a stroke. When Barbara developed some memory problems, she moved in with her daughter Diane. One morning, just after Barbara got up and entered the bathroom, she tripped and fell, hitting her head on the sink's granite counter. Diane rushed to the bathroom when she heard the thud. Barbara had a gash on her forehead, but she was conscious, and she seemed to be thinking and speaking coherently. Yet the next morning, Diane had to shake her mother to rouse her from sleep. When the paramedics arrived, Barbara was disoriented. By the time she got to the hospital, she could no longer speak.

Thirty-five-year-old Anita and her husband, Jeff, were going to the local Cinco de Mayo street fair with their two toddlers in tow. The crowd was thick, and as an unruly group of teenagers approached, the children walked closer to mom and dad. Then, in the blink of an eye, Anita was lying on the ground, groaning, while Jeff and the kids surrounded her. The details were hazy, but she remembered the teenagers pushing their way toward her just before it happened. After Anita hit the ground, she could not see clearly, and her heart raced. She touched her head and felt warm blood from her scalp. A bystander called to police as the crowd gradually dispersed. Anita tried to suppress the images that clouded her thinking as her husband helped her to her feet. The police arrived and took a report, after which the family went home, and all seemed well. But over the next few weeks, Anita started having headaches and more than her usual problems with insomnia.

Fifty-six-year-old Albert had always worked in a grocery store and gas station on the edge of his small town. With the economic downturn, times grew tougher, and he could no longer afford his medications for diabetes and high blood pressure. His life spiraled downward, and he lost his job and became homeless. The night the police raided his friend's house and arrested them for possessing crack cocaine, Albert hit bottom. He could not post bail, and the judge ordered a fifteen-year prison sentence. Albert had served a year when his nemesis, a fellow inmate, assaulted him in the yard. He awoke in solitary confinement with severe headaches.

Concussions can happen almost anywhere, not just during leisure activities or collision sports. In fact, simple falls, trauma from a blunt injury, or violent assault are the most frequent causes of a concussion or more serious TBI in the United States. Those most vulnerable to concussion are the very young, the very old, and society's most disadvantaged.

Younger Brains

Six large and flexible membranous areas of an infant's skull called fontanels or soft spots permit passage of the head through the birth canal and enable the brain to grow in utero. At birth, an infant's skull is composed of six separate bones—one frontal, one occipital, two parietal, and two temporal bones. During the first few years of life, these bones remain unfused, held together by cranial sutures (fibrous joints that have some elasticity). After birth, the cranial sutures and fontanels prevent the brain from compression as it develops and expands in size.

While the infant incurs benefits from her flexible skull, her head is particularly vulnerable to pressure and trauma. One example, plagiocephaly (flattening of the head), has become more common since the 1990s when the National Institutes of Health initiated the successful Back to Sleep Campaign to prevent sudden infant death syndrome (SIDS). Although infants should always be placed on their backs to sleep, only frequent repositioning and "tummy time" when awake can prevent plagiocephaly.

The anterior and largest fontanel is the last to close—it closes by the time a child reaches age 2. The fusing process of the cranial sutures occurs over multiple years as the brain continues to grow in size. Because a child's skull is particularly fragile during the first three years of life, parents must be vigilant to prevent head and brain injuries. Even up to age 5, children remain more vulnerable to brain injuries because their skulls have not fully hardened. A child's brain has a higher water content than an adult brain, and its axons are unmyelinated, so early childhood poses high risks for brain injury. Skull fractures in infants can result from what seem like minor falls from a low height, and children under the age of one obviously have a higher risk for injury than older children.

For infants and very young children, clinical diagnosis can be difficult. Usually there is swelling on the scalp from a bruise if the skull has been fractured. Because the skull fractures fairly easily in the young, there may be no obvious clinical signs of a brain injury such as loss of consciousness, a seizure, vomiting, lethargy, or irritability. In fact, these signs in infants can be hard to recognize because infants sleep much of the day, are naturally fussy, and spit up often, behaviors that would be worrisome in an adult who had hit her head. A fracture to the basilar skull (the bony base that the brain rests on) is even harder to diagnose in the very young. With more severe injuries, a child may show signs of bleeding around the orbits of the eyes ("raccoon eyes") or behind the ear (Battle's sign), and blood or fluid may also drain from the ear, just as occurs in adolescents and adults.

Young children are more likely to sustain injuries to the head from falling than older children or adults. Their centers of gravity are higher; they have less developed balance and coordination skills; their reaction time is slower; and they are more impulsive. Infants and young children are also more susceptible to TBIs than older children because their heads are larger relative to the rest of their bodies. The youngest children haven't developed the outstretched arm reflex that can cause wrist fractures but can spare the head.

Children often land headfirst when they fall, as Kali did. During growth spurts, the center of gravity changes, potentially impairing motor control and balance skills.

Kali's emergency room (ER) physician ordered a CT scan of her head because of the large bruise on her scalp, and the scan showed a small skull fracture, luckily not depressed into the brain, with no obvious brain bleeding or swelling. With some pain medication, Kali calmed down in a relatively quiet area of the ER. Intravenous fluids prevented the little girl from dehydrating while the staff closely monitored her, and she was admitted for a twenty-four-hour observation period. The next day, Kali went home with a follow-up appointment at her pediatrician's office a week later. She seemed to have recovered unscathed.

Diagnosing a concussion in a developing child can be a major challenge for physicians, because children may not be able to give information about their symptoms. The symptoms and signs of attention deficit disorder (ADD) and attention deficit hyperactivity disorder (ADHD) overlap with those of TBI, so concussions in young children may go unrecognized. Maya Evans, a pediatric physiatrist and specialist in brain injury medicine at the University of California, Davis, told me that "sometimes it is hard for parents and even health professionals to recognize that a pretty significant brain injury can exist when there is no visible injury seen on imaging studies, but a diagnosis can be made based on how the child is behaving in the minutes to days after the injury. We may see issues with learning and attention years later that may be the result of the injury. These skills are learned later and are the result of years of schooling and learning that require attention, focus and memory." Time would tell whether Kali's behaviors and learning would develop normally.

Equipment Dangers

Many product-related injuries occur from falls such as Kali's that involve impact to the head and neck, and concussions are the most common of these injuries. Busy parents like Stephanie may not buckle their child into a high chair, baby carrier, car seat, or stroller, or they may not use safety straps properly. Stephanie thought the tray on the high chair protected her daughter, so she did not buckle Kali in. Sadly, this is not unusual.

Infants placed on high surfaces, such as a changing table or really anywhere other than the floor, can fall in an instant once they begin to be able to reposition themselves. A high chair must have good stability and not sit near a wall or other piece of furniture that could topple the chair if the child kicks or pushes it. Not locking the wheels of a stroller or putting a bag on the handle in such a way that the stroller tips over can cause a fall and serious injury. Unanchored furniture or electronic equipment can topple when a curious child pulls it forward or climbs on it.

Parents and other caregivers are not always to blame. The leading category of children's products recalled in the United States are nursery products, and these products are found in households across the nation. The US Consumer Product Safety Commission tracks safety issues and product recalls for nursery equipment and furniture. Drop-side cribs were banned in the United States in 2011 because of high rates of injury after the side that releases was intentionally or unintentionally dropped and the child fell or jumped out. Walkers that enable babies to walk around with a set of rollers before they are developmentally capable of walking on their own can expose children to a number of hazards, including stairs. A campaign against these walkers has led to a decrease in injuries.

The Center for Injury Research and Policy (CIRP) at Nationwide Children's Hospital in Columbus, Ohio, tracks and researches safety in nursery products. The center reports that there are about 66,000 injuries annually related to these products, an underestimate because the study analyzed only emergency department data, and not all injuries lead to an ER visit. In one study of children's products, CIRP researchers found that two-thirds of injured children were not restrained or were climbing or standing in a high chair.

Christopher Gaw and his colleagues at CIRP conducted a study of approximately 1.3 million injuries related to nursery products among children less than 3 years old who were treated in ERs in the United States from 1991 to 2011. The injuries were most commonly associated with baby carriers, cribs, strollers, walkers, jumpers, or exercisers. The most common cause was a fall, and the most frequently injured body region was the head or neck. They saw a 34 percent decrease in the annual injury rate from 1991 to 2003, driven by a decline in injuries related to walkers, jumpers, or exercisers. However, concussions and closed head injuries (without skull fractures) increased by 24 percent from 2003 to 2011. Parents must be educated and vigilant about these potential dangers. Returning a completed manufacturer's product registration card helps to guarantee that they will be contacted if the product is recalled. CIRP also advises parents to read the manual and search for information about recalls.

Older Brains

By 2050, the population of those aged 65 years and older is expected to comprise about one-fifth of the total US population. By the same year, the global population of those aged 60 years and older is estimated to double from 900 million in 2015 to about 2 billion. Falls are the leading cause of fatal and nonfatal injuries among persons 65 years of age or older.

More than 80 percent of TBIs in adults aged 65 and older result from falls. In 2014, Gwen Bergen and other researchers at the Centers for Disease Control and Prevention (CDC) reported that 29 percent of older adults reported falling at least once in the preceding twelve months, resulting in an estimated 29 million falls that year. Of those who fell, nearly 38 percent reported at least one fall that required medical treatment or restricted their activity for at least a day. The total number for that year was a staggering 7 million fall injuries. Approximately half of older adults who fall do not discuss their falls with their health-care provider. The CDC emphasizes that providers can play an important role in fall prevention through risk screenings, avoiding medications linked to falls, and recommending vitamin D when appropriate for improved bone, muscle, and nerve health.

Older people like Barbara who have physical or cognitive disabilities are at the highest risks for falling. Barbara underwent emergency surgery to remove a subdural hematoma (SDH), a collection of blood under the dura, which is the hardest membrane covering the brain. Although Barbara did not lose consciousness when she fell, nor did she exhibit any other obvious sign of brain injury at first, her condition deteriorated overnight. The anticoagulant warfarin, a prescription medication Barbara had been taking, made her susceptible to bleeding when she fell. Barbara experienced a sequence typical in older patients. The absence of initial signs of a severe injury can lead to a false belief on the part of patients, families, and health-care providers that the injury is minor.

Older patients are at greater-than-average risk for SDHs because older brains can atrophy (shrink), leading to stretching and rupturing of the blood vessels called bridging veins. A brain bleed may

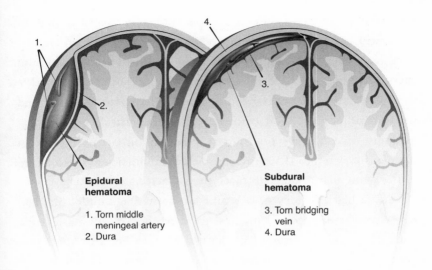

Epidural hematoma

1. Torn middle meningeal artery
2. Dura

Subdural hematoma

3. Torn bridging vein
4. Dura

FIGURE 8 Two major types of cerebral bleeding: subdural and epidural hematomas.

then occur with very minor or even no apparent trauma. A blow to the head injuring the middle meningeal artery can cause another type of bleeding called an epidural hematoma (EDH). An EDH or SDH can expand quickly, leading to pressure on the brain. Hernia-tion (squeezing or pushing part of the brain) through the foramen magnum (the hole at the base of the skull) causes pressure on respi-ratory and other vital systems in the brainstem. Death follows unless a craniotomy (opening of the skull) relieves the pressure and the blood is evacuated (removed) (see Figure 8).

Intimate Partner Violence

Intimate partner violence (IPV) is a significant cause of TBI. The CDC defines IPV as physical, emotional, or sexual harm by a former or current partner or spouse. It disproportionately affects women. In fact, estimates are that approximately 25 percent of women experience physical IPV during their lifetime, making it more common than breast cancer, diabetes, and depression combined. Many IPV survivors have experienced a TBI because blows to the head and neck are among the most common types of injuries. Harvard psychologist Eve Valera's preliminary research on brain injuries in women subjected to IPV provides scientific evidence of the damage to the white matter (axonal tracts) they experience.

Anita had a history of IPV and was abused as a child. She had never sought or received medical care for these traumatic events. This is common among IPV victims. During her first marriage, Anita's husband often punched her in the face, shoved her against the wall, or threw her to the floor when he got angry. She went to the ER once or twice with a black eye, but no one ever asked about IPV, and she was too embarrassed to bring it up. Some people with concussions are less likely to seek treatment or go to ERs than those with more visible injuries because they perceive their injuries as not life-threatening. IPV victims are even less likely to seek treatment because they feel shame or fear. Studies suggest that health-care providers only identify 3 to 10 percent of victims, even when victims do seek care for injuries.

As it turned out, although Anita fell and hit her head at the street fair and had a scalp injury, she did not receive a concussion there. She remembered events before and after the incident. Instead, she was diagnosed with post-traumatic stress disorder (PTSD) and severe, untreated depression. When she fell, Anita experienced flashbacks to decades of child abuse and IPV. People with a history of experiencing or witnessing traumatic events can suppress those images, only to have them emerge later when another disturbing or traumatic event occurs.

What Anita experienced is known as an abreaction, the release of emotional tension as a result of a trigger in the person's environment. That trigger can be a spoken word or phrase, the closeness of a strange crowd, a period of complete aloneness, a darkened room, or a sensation such as smell, touch, or sound associated with the original trauma. The trigger can unwillingly and unknowingly transport the person back to the time of the original event, causing them to react in the current moment with what was appropriate emotional intensity at that previous traumatic moment. A person experiencing an abreaction can actually have trouble distinguishing between the past and present.

Anita's headaches and insomnia resolved after successful treatment for PTSD and depression. Her second husband devotedly helped her through the recovery process. Internist Brigid McCaw, IPV expert and former·medical director of the Kaiser Permanente Family Violence Prevention Program, pointed out to me that "Contrary to many people's impressions, most women end abusive relationships and do not go on to have other abusive relationships. However, there can be health effects that can be long lasting." This was the case with Anita.

Child Abuse

Nonaccidental injuries to very young children due to child abuse go by various names, with shaken baby syndrome (SBS) the term most often used in the media. SBS implies that the brain injury occurs when a parent or caregiver shakes a crying baby out of frustration or anger. Diagnosis has primarily rested on three findings: brain swelling, a SDH identified on imaging studies, and bleeding in the retina (back of the eye) diagnosed by an eye examination. Controversies about the SBS diagnosis have swirled around medical and legal spheres for decades. US courts have overturned convictions, and scientists even debate whether SBS is due to shaking at all, because some cases may be related to birth trauma, falls, or assaults that do not involve shaking.

Today pediatric abusive head trauma (AHT) is the preferred term, because shaking is not the only cause of injury to the head and brain, and of course babies are not the only children or adolescents who suffer abuse from caregivers. Punching, kicking, or striking the head or dropping, throwing, suffocation, or shaking can lead to swelling and bleeding in the brain or other injuries that result in death or disability. Child abuse is often unreported for obvious reasons: babies cannot talk, children may fear retaliation or lack the ability to find help and communicate with adults outside the home, and visible signs of injury may be lacking.

When an infant or child has an injury to the brain or skull, a pattern of swelling, SDH, and retinal hemorrhages strongly suggests pediatric AHT. The diagnosis is based on gathering more information from adults and observing other signs of trauma. Infants and children who survive may be left with a variety of lifelong challenges, including learning disabilities, seizures, paralysis, and blindness or other disabling conditions. Even a concussion, without major findings on neuroimaging studies, can cause permanent changes in personality, behavior, and cognitive function.

In 2014, the National Child Abuse and Neglect Data System (NCANDS) reported that there were 702,000 victims of child abuse and neglect in the United States. The most vulnerable are the youngest children—those younger than 5 years and, particularly, infants younger than 1 year. Eighty percent of perpetrators are parents, and most perpetrators are male. Child abusers are most often the father, stepfather, the mother's boyfriend, a babysitter, or the mother. The victimization rate has been slightly higher for girls, but the fatality rate is higher among abused boys.

Child abuse has been identified as the cause of TBI in 25 percent of children older than 2. Assault is the leading cause of TBI-related death among infants and children up to age 4, accounting for approximately 40 percent of deaths in this age category. The CDC reported 2,250 deaths of children under age 5 from AHT between 1999 and 2014. Fortunately, that same report found that rates declined in the second half of the study period. Child abuse numbers are conservative because they include only cases where the injury was recognized by a provider and recorded and classified as an assault. It's possible that many abuse-related TBIs in children are either missed completely, misclassified, or not classified because the child is treated in a setting where data is not collected or accurately coded.

The ER physician and the social worker both had lots of questions about Kali's fall from the high chair. They were aware that caregivers rarely admit abusing infants and children and frequently report that the child fell out of a crib, bed, or high chair, or else fell down a set of stairs. However, Kali's mother, Stephanie, was not evasive, and the information she provided about what happened was consistent and credible. She was contrite about not securing Kali into the chair with the safety harness.

Kali's CT scan showed just one undepressed fracture in the frontal bone, and there was no evidence of contusions (bruising), brain lacerations (tears), or SDH. The physician knew that a bleed in the brain was much less likely to occur from a short fall. Her examination did not uncover any other signs of injury such as bruising, rib or long bone fractures, neck injuries, or retinal hemorrhages. The nurse, social worker, and physician educated Stephanie about providing a safe environment for her child and always using baby products with safety in mind. Stephanie also received information about tip-over risks of furniture, televisions, and other household objects before she took Kali home.

Elder Abuse

Similarly, the physician and social worker posed many questions to Diane about her mother Barbara's fall in the bathroom. Diane's great concern about her mother, her regret that she did not bring her in for an evaluation immediately after the fall, and her answers to questions about the circumstances of the injury convinced these healthcare professionals that no abuse had occurred. On Barbara's physical examination, there were no signs of self-defense injuries, such as bruises on her arms.

Elder abuse is rising in incidence as the US baby boomer population ages. Estimates are that one in ten seniors experiences some form of elder abuse every month in the United States and across the globe. This translates to an annual estimated 5 million older Americans suffering elder abuse, neglect, or exploitation. This is an underestimate, because like child abuse or IPV, only a small fraction of cases are reported to authorities. Those most at risk are elderly women, people with dementia, mental illness, or multiple physical illnesses, elders living with adult children, and elders with lower socioeconomic status. Elderly patients with Alzheimer's disease are five times more likely to experience abuse than other elders.

Seniors are susceptible to physical, financial, sexual, and emotional abuse or neglect. Elderly poly-victimization (when two or more forms of abuse occur concurrently) affects from one in ten to one in twelve seniors internationally. A senior's primary caregiver, frequently the patient's spouse or adult child, is most likely to be the abuser. Abusers are also more likely to be male and to have a mental health condition or a history of substance abuse. Unemployed caregivers under financial stress or who are socially isolated also have a greater likelihood of becoming abusive.

Prisons and Homelessness

Albert was one of about 2 million people, mostly men, who reside in US prisons and jails. Many like Albert are men of color, caught in a punitive and systemically discriminatory justice system. The US incarceration rate increased 500 percent over the last four decades (although there has been a slight decline annually since 2007). In a range of studies, 25 percent to 87 percent of prison inmates report having experienced a head injury or TBI, compared to 8.5 percent of the general population. Albert had been convicted of a nonviolent crime, as are many prisoners in the United States. Like many prisoners, he had a history of depression and substance use. As a homeless person prior to prison, Albert's risk of a TBI was also very high.

There is more research in Canada than in the United States or other countries exploring the associations of TBI and homelessness. In one Canadian study, Jane Topolovec-Vranic and her co-investigators found that more than half of a group of homeless people had a history of a TBI with loss of consciousness. This association raises the odds of depression, other mood disorders, and PTSD, just as being incarcerated does. In another Canadian study by Tomislov Svoboda and Jason Ramsey, homeless men were estimated to have rates of head injury that were fourteen times higher than those in the general population of Canada, with a rate 400 times higher among those who were chronically homeless with drinking problems.

Albert's altercation with another prisoner raises the possibility that he had problems controlling his anger and may have been impulsive or disinhibited before the injury. If so, this may have resulted from an undiagnosed TBI. Seema Fazel and colleagues conducted a large population study using a Swedish national registry and found that approximately 9 percent of people with a history of TBI had committed violent crimes. This contrasted with a rate of 2 to 3 percent in the population control group. There was some weakening of the association of TBI and violent crime when familial factors and substance abuse were added into the analysis.

This link between TBI and crime also appeared in studies conducted by Australian and Canadian researchers. Psychologist W. Huw Williams and co-authors summarized this research: "these studies indicate that TBI is an independent risk factor for crime. In the very young, it could lead to later drug and alcohol misuse, which, in turn, increases likelihood of crime. In those injured after 5 years of age, including adults, TBI appears to be linked to increased likelihood of offending . . . . TBI could add to greater risk of criminality by increasing likelihood of problem behaviour and eroding capacity for self-regulation and socialisation."

TBI interrelates with many other factors that have yet to be fully explored in research studies. Since Albert lost consciousness during the incident and became conscious only when he was already in solitary confinement, the circumstances leading up to the incident remain unclear. The CDC points out that attention and memory problems after a TBI may be misread by corrections officers as a lack of cooperation or defiance, something that can lead to disciplinary actions.

Some Years Later

When Kali reached first grade and a developmental pediatrician diagnosed her as having ADHD, Stephanie wondered if there was a connection to the concussion Kali had had at age 2. Children who have had a concussion before the age of 5 are more likely to show symptoms of ADHD, conduct disorder, or oppositional defiant behavior, substance use disorder, and mood disorder when they reach adolescence, so that was a possibility.

After Barbara's surgery, she was discharged to an inpatient rehabilitation program for three weeks. The attending physiatrist let Diane know that her mother was at high risk for another injury from a fall in the years to come because she had difficulties with walking as well as balance and vision problems. The physiatrist was careful not to overtreat Barbara's hypertension, and she avoided giving her any tranquilizers or sedatives. Physical therapy provided her with a walker, and the physician ordered home health physical and occupational therapy and a shower chair. The social worker had provided Diane with the CDC's web address and a STEADI (Stopping Elderly Accidents, Deaths, and Injuries) packet of materials.

When Barbara saw her primary care physician one week after her discharge from the rehabilitation hospital, he recommended cataract surgery for both eyes. After the cataract surgery, Barbara's ophthalmologist advised her to stop wearing progressive lenses, because they confused her when she looked down while walking or going down stairs. Diane installed a railing at the front door of the house and an additional railing on the inside stairs, removed the throw rugs and clutter around the house, installed a toilet surround and grab bars for the shower, and had an electrician assess the house for improved lighting and installation of motion sensors. Barbara walked at home and outdoors with a walker and needed only minimal assistance for self-care. What began as mild memory issues, however, accelerated into dementia over the next few years. When Barbara fell in the shower, her daughter placed her in a long-term care facility near their home. Two years later, she died under hospice care.

Anita was successfully treated with an antidepressant and cognitive-behavioral therapy (CBT). The psychotherapist used a specific technique called eye movement desensitization reprocessing (EMDR). EMDR involves the use of a hand-motion technique to guide a patient's eye movements while the patient watches a pendulum swing. It is not clear how the treatment works, but it has achieved success in some patients with PTSD, anxiety, phobias, and other mental health disorders. As Anita's mood improved and her PTSD symptoms waned, she found more and more pleasure in life, especially in taking care of her family.

Albert's TBI was not diagnosed or appropriately treated while he was in prison, although he received substance abuse treatment during incarceration. The CDC, criminal justice professionals, and TBI experts have recommended that prisoners with a history of TBI, mental health, and / or substance abuse problems be assigned case managers who can coordinate placement in community treatment programs upon their release from prison. Unfortunately, Albert received no transition services during his community re-entry.

Albert was released from prison after five years of incarceration. He found help through a Medicaid health-care plan once he was on parole. He finally was able to get a comprehensive evaluation at our rehabilitation center. I referred him for a neuropsychological evaluation that revealed that he had not only a TBI and post-traumatic headaches, but depression and PTSD. Treatment for all of his diagnoses resulted in an excellent recovery. While on disability, he took care of his elderly mother, who was dying of metastatic breast cancer.

Long-Term Outcomes

Large population studies can provide a broader view of how a concussion might contribute to or be associated with other psychiatric or medical problems later in life. Often these studies are done in countries that have large population health research databases, and where people and their outcomes are easier to track over time.

In a Swedish registry study, Amir Sariaslan, David Sharp, Seena Fazel, and their co-investigators mined data from the records of

1.1 million individuals born between 1973 and 1985, to research children and adolescents who experienced at least one brain injury. They wondered if TBI in young people was associated with significant medical and social problems in adulthood. They used a case-control approach and compared outcomes with unaffected siblings. Seventy-five percent of the group had suffered a mild TBI. They found a connection between all severities of TBI and subsequent psychiatric visits, inpatient hospitalizations, premature mortality, low educational attainment, and receipt of disability pensions and welfare benefits.

The researchers found that recurring injuries, such as multiple sports concussions, increased the likelihood of one or more of these poorer outcomes. Older age at first injury, especially after age 15, increased the risk of worse outcomes. For example, there was less likelihood of a bad outcome if the first injury occurred before age 4 as opposed to an injury occurring between ages 20 and 24. This may suggest that the very young brain may recover more easily, but we can't reach firm conclusions.

Is a seizure disorder or epilepsy (two or more seizures occurring over time) a risk after a concussion? The research is conflicting. Canadian researcher Richard Wennberg and his colleagues concluded that a group of 330 patients (average age 28) with mild TBIs did not have a significant risk of epilepsy over a five- to ten-year period. On the other hand, Jakob Christensen and fellow researchers used a much larger Danish population database and found the risk of epilepsy to be about two times greater in children with mild TBI than in those without that history. The risk was highest during the first year after the injury and decreased over time. Not surprisingly, genetic susceptibility emerged as a key factor. At ten years, the risk was still higher for children with mild TBI and a family history of epilepsy.

The association of TBI and neurodegenerative conditions, including dementia, is documented in many studies (see Chapter 4). Recurrent injuries after a TBI are a risk, especially in the elderly. Kristen Dams-O'Connor of the Mount Sinai School of Medicine collaborated with researchers from the Adult Changes in Thought research group (a Kaiser Permanente Washington Health Research Institute and University of Washington collaboration) to track and assess risk of injury and death for those age 65 or older who had a history of a TBI. No association was found for subsequent death, but there was a risk of subsequent injury, particularly in those 55 or older at the time of the TBI, during the period under study (an average of seven years).

Observational studies raise the question of reverse causality. In other words, do genetic factors, social determinants of health, or other unmeasured factors in these studies predispose a person to these outcomes? Much more research is needed to understand the risks for and outcomes after a concussion in children, adolescents, and adults. While the individual stories of Kali, Barbara, Anita, and Albert are compelling and relatable, they are unique and cannot be used to predict outcomes for other children or adults with these types of injuries.

A Link to the Next Chapter

Warfare always carries a major risk of concussion and more severe TBIs, as we will see in the last chapter. Although women bear similar risks to men in combat, women in the military may have other risks for TBI. Philadelphia Veterans Administration (VA) social worker Melissa Dichter and her colleagues found in their research that one-third of veteran women reported a history of IPV at some point in their lives, compared with about one-fourth of women who had not served in the military. Clinical psychologist Katherine

Iverson also investigates the connection between IPV-related TBI through her work at the Women's Health Sciences Division of the VA's National Center for PTSD. Iverson and her colleagues found, not unexpectedly, that IPV-related TBI is associated with poorer mental and physical health in women veterans, and she explores treatments that lead to the best outcomes. Her research is a reminder that there are many interrelationships in concussion risks and outcomes for vulnerable people and populations, but also that there are treatments.

9

War and Work

As a lieutenant in the US Army, my patient Jamie saw his share of combat during his deployment to Afghanistan. Jamie had seen soldiers suffer major injuries and become permanently disfigured or disabled. Many died. He'd also seen soldiers suffer concussions from roadside explosions, only to get up after the initial shock, shake off the dirt, and feel better in a few weeks without medical intervention. One day while off base near Kandahar in his Humvee, a roadside bomb exploded a couple of yards away. The blast force threw Jamie from his vehicle, and he landed in a pile of rubble. He doesn't remember exactly what he was doing when he lost consciousness or how long he was out, but he awakened on the ground. The medics found him dizzy, confused, and complaining of a headache. Jamie suffered both a blast injury and blunt injuries from the explosion.

Jamie was initially evaluated using military neurocognitive assessment tests (NCATs; see Chapter 2 for more discussion of these tests). The assessments suggested significant problems with attention and memory. The military uses a number of NCATs, including the Military Acute Concussion Evaluation (MACE), to evaluate military personnel suspected of a concussion or more severe brain injury during combat or while deployed in a war zone. Military specialty clinics then administer the Automated Neuropsychological Assessment Metrics (ANAM) and the Defense Automated Neurobehavioral Assessment (DANA) to further assess injured soldiers. Jamie's results helped to determine that he needed more extensive evaluations, and he returned to the United States to receive care through the Veterans Administration system.

Soldiers have always risked TBIs during wartime, and nothing equals the combat theater for a high-risk environment. The term "theater" seems appropriate, given the drama, angst, pathos, and trauma of wartime. TBI risk was already extremely high during the two world wars, and it has risen exponentially in the late twentieth and early twenty-first centuries as armed conflicts expand in number and intensity. It seems there is always a war going on someplace in the world.

Blast Waves and Winds

A blast wave is produced by a collection of gases that advance outward at a speed faster than sound. The blast initially exerts a positive pressure, but its primary effect comes from the shock wave that follows, and then from a blast wind. A blast from an improvised explosive device, land mine, rocket grenade, or other device can cause a TBI in a number of ways. Shock waves may create a pressure vacuum and cause violent shaking. Flying shrapnel or other objects may hit military personnel, who might also be thrown against or onto a hard surface. Thermal (heat), chemical, and other injuries to the head, including the face, scalp, and respiratory tract, may cause additional injury. When a blast hits someone riding in a vehicle, injuries can occur from the initial shock wave or from a projectile. The force of a blast is always more intense in an enclosed setting, such as a vehicle or a building. In Jamie's case, all of these injury mechanisms were at work. Blast waves can also reflect off surfaces and become more complex. Mach stem formation refers to the reflection of a blast wave off the ground, after which the wave joins with the original shock front to create even higher pressures.

Researchers theorize that blast wave energy enters the brain and other parts of the body in a split second through vulnerable openings such as eye sockets, ears, nose, and mouth, or through the circulatory or respiratory system. For example, surges of blood or an air embolism (a bubble of air that travels through the circulatory system) can produce vascular injuries, such as a stroke. Figure 9 shows the various entry points where a blast wave may enter.

More prolonged cerebral edema (brain swelling) and vasospasm (closing off of blood vessels) seems to occur more often in blast TBIs than in blunt TBIs. Fluids and solids in the brain respond differently to a shock wave than to a blunt force impact. These waves produce rapid pressure changes that injure organs that contain a combination of air and fluids, such as the stomach and bladder. If forceful enough, the waves may penetrate the skull and travel through the large blood vessels in the chest and abdomen. Blast waves also create a greater likelihood of additional injuries to the eyes, ears, the vestibular system, and the pituitary gland. A study by David Baxter and colleagues from the United Kingdom showed that one out of every three soldiers with a blast injury has pituitary hormone abnormalities, such as low thyroid or growth hormone.

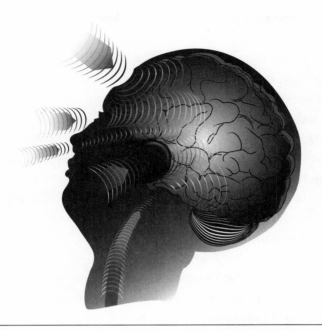

FIGURE 9 Entry points for blast wave energy causing a brain injury.

Blast waves can cause brain injuries similar to those caused by acceleration-deceleration forces. Cellular events such as diffuse axonal injury (DAI), microvascular damage (blood-vessel damage), neuroinflammation, microglia activation, and elevations in phosphorylated tau (p-tau) can occur from blasts. White matter tracts are at least as vulnerable in blast TBI as in other types of TBI. In one MRI study of veterans exposed to blasts, half had scans showing injury to axonal tracts such as the cingulate cortex and the corpus callosum (see Chapter 1). Pathologists Sharon Shively and Daniel Perl from the Center for Neuroscience and Regenerative Medicine's Brain Tissue Repository at the Uniformed Services University in Bethesda, Maryland, reported gliosis (reaction of the glial cells to trauma that can result in scarring) at gray-white matter junctions and within the structures that line the fluid-filled ventricles of the brain.

The axonal pattern of injury after a blast may differ from that caused by other forces. A group of scientists at the 2015 International State-of-the-Science meeting, sponsored by the Department of Defense, concluded that DAI did not seem to be a characteristic of blast injuries. However, neuropsychologist Jasmeet Hayes and her Boston colleagues found evidence of white matter tract changes using diffusion tensor imaging (DTI) in veterans with blast injuries, and Canadian researcher Eugene Park and his colleagues demonstrated axonal injury after a blast exposure in laboratory models. (See Chapter 1 for more discussion of axons, glial cells, gray and white matter, DAI, white matter tracts, and DTI.)

Studies show that blast and blunt TBI groups have similar rates of pain, vision loss, vestibular dysfunction, depression, sleep disorders, other post-concussion symptoms, and other day-to-day challenges. Care and treatment for these patients primarily entails educating them and providing symptom management strategies (see Chapter 3). However, individualized treatment must be based on the unique aspects of military injuries.

Existing population studies have not yet clarified the true incidence and prevalence of blast-related injuries in US military personnel. Many of these studies do not report how long it takes from the time of the blast to a medical assessment. Of those that do report this interval, most find assessments taking place only after thirty days to a year from the time of the blast exposure. A failure of systems within the military sometimes creates this delay, and in other cases the delay is due to a lack of reporting by service men and women.

As blast injuries have increased in number, so too have advances in medical care, safety measures, and protective equipment that have improved survival odds. Here's a cruel irony, however: a soldier wearing protective gear such as body armor is less vulnerable to lung and heart trauma but has a greater chance of surviving with the consequences of a blast injury to the brain. Like athletes who wear protective gear to play collision sports, service members may experience repeated low-level blasts that are a common feature of war zones and that, cumulatively, may lead to devastating brain injuries.

Wars Past

Frederick Mott, a practicing physician and pathologist at the Maudsley Hospital in London during World War I, autopsied the brains of soldiers diagnosed with shell shock after being exposed to explosions, and he found damage in the corpus callosum. Mott also investigated concussion's possible hormonal and other physical effects, and he identified chronic symptoms that he ascribed to the brain's vulnerability following concussions. He used the term *locus minoris resistentiae*—loosely translated as a place of less resistance to disease or injury, an Achilles heel. Physicians in other branches of medicine have used this term to explain, for example, why cancer may occur in a cirrhotic liver or in an osteoporotic limb, or why infection takes root in a damaged heart valve. Mott made the point that a concussed brain becomes less resistant to the effects of another concussion, which he observed in wounded soldiers he treated at Maudsley.

During the Civil War, the walking wounded who displayed cognitive, behavioral, and mood disturbances of war were said to have a soldier's heart, a reference to the psychological effects of trauma. During World War I, when explosive shelling during intense trench warfare caused TBIs, the term shell shock described a blast injury that did not entail overt signs of trauma to the head or brain but was accompanied by a range of symptoms and behaviors of psychic, if not physical, trauma. Intense trench warfare with the use of explosive devices brought multiple trauma to a horrific new level. Another term—combat stress reaction—denoted something akin to post-traumatic stress disorder (PTSD), a diagnosis that emerged only in the 1970s during the Vietnam War.

Medical historian Stephen Casper stresses in his book *The Neurologists* that physicians in the emerging specialty became the first experts at addressing the complex diagnosis of shell shock. Neurologists were trained to diagnose both physical and psychological disorders, and their medical specialty often was asked to determine who was malingering or attempting to avoid going back into combat. In 1922, the British War Office convened the Southborough Commission, a group of physicians and other experts who interviewed injured soldiers with a history of the disorder labeled shell shock. Ultimately the term was abandoned because it lacked precision.

By 1939, about 120,000 British World War I veterans had received final awards for a disability. Although the word had fallen into disfavor, shell shock stirred debate in the medical and psychological discourse of World War II and beyond. People still primarily ascribed the prolonged symptoms and behaviors of veterans to a wounding of the psyche rather than the brain. Terms such as war neurosis, hysteria, and neurasthenia reflected this "it's all in your mind" conclusion. Lieutenant Colonel Roy R. Grinker and Captain John P. Spiegel acknowledged both the physical and psychological effects of concussion in their 1943 monograph, *War Neuroses in North Africa,* but they ultimately placed psychological scars above physical ones:

> When fatigue, hunger and thirst are combined with continuous exposure to danger and the constant pounding of heavy artillery and serial bombs, the resistance of even the strongest to the development of anxiety may become impaired.

The purely physiological effects of a nearby blast are also a factor. Many men are repeatedly subjected to minimal doses of blast. They are knocked over by the compression wave, or perhaps blown slightly off the ground, if they are lying prone. In some instances, they are temporarily numbed or even stunned. Such injuries are not to be interpreted as responsible for the symptoms which occur in the neurosis; but merely as one of the factors responsible for the general reduction of the ego's capacity to resist anxiety.

The words used to express the psychological aspects of these World War II injuries—anxiety, neurosis, hysteria, and reduction of ego capacity—reflect the influence of psychodynamic theories still in vogue during that era. Grinker trained in neurology and psychiatry, and Sigmund Freud was among his mentors. Grinker and Spiegel both practiced as psychiatrists, not neurologists.

In 1980, the American Psychiatric Association added PTSD to the third edition of its *Diagnostic and Statistical Manual of Mental Disorders* (DSM-III). This addition reflected not only new terminology but also new concepts and requirements for diagnosis. A PTSD diagnosis required symptoms and behaviors to result from a traumatic event, not a neurosis. But as is clear, the TBI-PTSD mystery remains unsolved, and a new term—polytrauma—has now surfaced.

The Polytrauma Debates

Today, the word trauma holds different meanings depending on whether it is applied to mental or physical conditions. We now live in a post-Freudian era that takes anatomic and physiologic explanations more seriously. However, the mental versus physical debates have continued among clinicians. In 2008, Charles Hoge, a psychiatrist at the Walter Reed Army Institute of Research, and his colleagues published results of a study of US soldiers in Iraq in which 44 percent of those reporting a mild TBI with loss of consciousness met criteria for PTSD, and 27 percent of those with altered mental status (but not loss of consciousness) met PTSD criteria. Soldiers with mild TBI were significantly more likely to report poor general health, missed workdays, medical visits, and more post-concussion and physical symptoms than those with other injuries. Hoge and colleagues concluded that, after adjusting for PTSD and depression, TBI in the veterans he studied was no longer associated with physical health symptoms (including post-concussion symptoms), except for headache.

Hoge's research and additional commentary in 2009 in the *New England Journal of Medicine* clearly resurfaced the debates. In an editorial accompanying the article, psychologist Richard A. Bryant agreed that the research substantiates the view that symptoms after a concussion are primarily, if not exclusively, due to psychological phenomena. On the other hand, he stated that "neural networks involve the regulation of anxiety" and these networks might be injured. He also speculated that perhaps cognitive reserve (a person's capacity to maintain cognitive function even with brain pathology) might be inadequate and therefore might explain cognitive symptoms. He concluded that diagnosis is difficult, and he predicted: "If troops currently serving in Iraq or Afghanistan are informed about a postconcussive syndrome and persistent problems emerging from mild traumatic brain injury, a new syndrome could arise from the current conflict in which soldiers attribute a range of common stress reactions to the effects of brain injury. This could be damaging to morale and to the person's future mental health, because it could lead to the expectation of poor recovery."

Letters to the editor followed Hoge's articles and Bryant's commentary. Researchers and clinicians questioned Hoge's research methods—information collected long after trauma exposure, a lack of information about pre-injury psychiatric conditions, and inadequate examinations that could have identified other medical conditions. Physiatrists argued for an interdisciplinary approach that follows Veterans Administration (VA) guidelines and identifies the physical and psychological conditions and comprehensive treatment found in rehabilitation medicine clinics within the VA. Such approaches need not be limited, they argued, to treating PTSD, depression, or other psychological conditions. They pushed for treatment strategies for chronic pain, substance abuse, other medical problems, and health education. This approach characterizes the new polytrauma approach.

A related study by VA physiatrist David Cifu and his colleagues, with more than 600,000 returning combatants from the Operation Enduring Freedom (OEF) conflict in Afghanistan and the Operation Iraqi Freedom (OIF) and Operation New Dawn (OND) conflicts, determined that over half of injured soldiers had one or more of a triad of diagnoses: TBI, PTSD, and pain. About 40 percent received a pain diagnosis, 30 percent had PTSD, and 10 percent had a TBI diagnosis, with about 6 percent diagnosed with all three conditions. It has always been difficult to discern when a soldier's symptoms result from a TBI and when they form part of a mood disorder or a painful condition.

David Cifu explained to me how current language expresses this complexity and the problem of inadequate diagnosis:

Each war brings concussive injuries to men and women in combat, whether from mace blows to metal helmets, cannons pulled by horse carts, or IEDs. These injuries are exacerbated and complicated by the physical and emotional horrors of battle. These polytrauma injuries are frequently overlooked, underdiagnosed, or mislabeled, but they clearly begin with mild physical trauma resulting in a classic brain injury from acceleration–deceleration and rotational forces. Polytrauma injuries are compounded by the pre- and post-injury stressors of war, such as poor nutrition, insomnia, anxiety, and fear produced by life and death situations. Undertreatment of somatic issues, such as pain and dizziness, leads to an array of problems variably attributed to blast, toxins, environmental issues, and other often nebulous factors.

A comprehensive polytrauma approach to diagnosis and treatment will no doubt lead to the best outcomes for soldiers and veterans like Jamie. Jamie served in the army for five years and deployed to Iraq and Afghanistan three times. In the days following his concussion, Jamie continued to work in spite of headaches, ringing in his ears, dizziness, and fatigue. Because he wanted a long-term career in the army, he refused to give in to his symptoms. As he struggled with remembering appointments and other details, the stigma of a mental health diagnosis haunted him. Nightmares plagued his sleep, and he got little more than a few hours rest each night. During the day, he tried to keep busy and not think about the explosion or his buddies who had recovered from injuries like his within weeks and without taking a medical leave. Why did he continue to struggle?

When the blast occurred outside Jamie's Humvee, the trauma transported him to several years earlier when an IED had decapitated his friend Howard. Jamie reacted to his own injury with the same emotional intensity he experienced when Howard died. Jamie felt the blast that killed Howard, but because he was more than 165 feet from the explosion and didn't have any blast-related symptoms, he was not given the mandatory medical examination that follows a

blast experience. But Jamie had recurrent thoughts and visions related to that horrible day. The abreactions—a releasing of emotional
tension as a result of environmental triggers—resembled Anita's reexperiencing of child abuse and intimate partner violence when she
was injured (see Chapter 8).

A person suffering from PTSD reexperiences the traumatic
event, avoids situations that provoke a reexperiencing, demonstrates
hypervigilance and heightened startle reflexes, and has nightmares
and flashbacks that disrupt sleep and concentration. These symptoms and behaviors do not characterize concussions or more severe
TBIs. Only an experienced clinician with adequate time and the
opportunity to establish trust and rapport with the injured individual can make this distinction.

While cognitive problems, such as memory difficulties or slow
information processing, usually result from an injury to the brain
rather than from a psychic trauma, they may also accompany chronic
insomnia, chronic pain, anxiety, and other co-morbidities that
occur with trauma exposure, especially exposure associated with
PTSD. At the same time, depression, substance abuse, and suicide
link to both PTSD and TBI. These difficulties often lead to lifelong problems that affect a person's ability to work and maintain a
stable family life. Christine MacDonald's group of Department of
Defense researchers found concussive blast TBI to be associated
with worsening rather than improving PTSD and depression
symptoms over a five-year period. However, the analyses did not
include data about this group's access to and use of mental health
care.

Conventional wisdom used to hold that a concussion or more
severe TBI involving loss of consciousness protected the injured
person from PTSD because he or she would not remember what had
happened. However, a number of studies suggest that the risk of

PTSD is actually heightened when a TBI occurs. A study led by biomedical engineer Tim Walilko of Oklahoma City bombing survivors showed a significant association between TBI and PTSD, but not PTSD and other injuries.

We are not sure what these findings linking TBI and PTSD mean. Could physical trauma to the brain cause or contribute to PTSD? Is there a common brain structure that is malfunctioning in both TBI and PTSD? Some MRI studies suggest that the structures functioning abnormally in PTSD—the amygdala, the area of the brain that processes emotions, particularly fear; the hippocampus, an area responsible for the formation of memory; and the orbito-frontal cortex, which controls attention span and emotions—are the same areas of the brain most likely to malfunction after a TBI, including a blast TBI.

Cyrus Raji, a researcher at the University of California, Los Angeles, and his co-investigators have used imaging studies to investigate differences in blood flow in the default mode network (DMN) in PTSD and TBI patients. This network links the orbito-frontal cortex, the hippocampus, and the cingulate cortex. Patients with PTSD showed evidence of increased blood flow, and those with TBI showed decreased blood flow. Other MRI studies have not found differences between the brains of veterans with PTSD and those without PTSD, so the jury is still out on the brain differences question for PTSD and TBI.

A Suicide Epidemic?

Suicide has been identified as a risk for people with concussion in noncombat settings. Seena Fazel's large Swedish registry study of premature death for people with a history of TBI revealed a twofold higher risk of premature death from injury, suicide, assault, or other causes for people with a history of mild TBI when compared with a general population. University of Toronto's Michael Fralick and co-investigators conducted a systematic review of ten studies of the association of suicide and concussion. They found there was twice the risk of suicide for people with a history of concussion compared to those without a history of concussion.

The risks for military men and women are even greater. A history of TBI means a higher risk for PTSD, depression, and suicidal thoughts and behaviors. The Department of Veterans Affairs reports about twenty suicide deaths every day among veterans, about one and a half times more often than those who have not served in the military. That amounts to 6,132 veterans and 1,387 servicemembers who died by suicide in one year. We may not always be able to connect the suicide of an individual to a concussion or to repeated concussions. However, suicide prevention is a necessary part of any comprehensive treatment program for people with TBI, especially for military personnel.

New York Times journalist Jennifer Steinhauer summarized the problem of veteran and civilian suicides this way: "While the V.A. has been the public face of the issue, veterans are in many ways an amplification of the same factors that drive suicide in the broader American population: a fragmented healthcare system, a shortage of mental health resources, especially in rural areas, a lack of funding for suicide research and easy access to guns. All of these contribute to the drastically increased suicide rate among all Americans, which rose 33 percent from 1999 to 2017."

Health Care for Military Personnel

The Veterans Administration and the Department of Defense established TBI rehabilitation services, programs, and related research gradually. VA physiatrist David Cifu and his co-authors document this evolution, pointing out that the establishment of the Defense and Veterans Head Injury Program in 1992 (now the Defense and Veterans Brain Injury Center or DVBIC) represented a historic watershed. The DVBIC led the way in establishing standards of evaluation and treatment for TBI, as well as developing instruments such as the MACE to detect milder TBIs (see Chapter 2). Care of soldiers and veterans, if comprehensive and individualized, can be effective when individuals have access to it. I asked David Cifu to sum it up, and he put it this way: "The research has consistently demonstrated that the only causes that support the persistent symptoms and difficulties of service members and veterans are mild TBI with concomitant psychological conditions such as PTSD, anxiety, depression, and pain. The existing treatments for these complicated mild TBI's work quite well when delivered in a holistic and patient-centered manner."

Commanders are required to evaluate any service member exposed to a blow to the head or a blast, either in a vehicle or other enclosed space, or at a certain distance from the explosion. If any injury occurs with a witnessed loss of consciousness, an evaluation is mandatory. Current VA policy requires that all OEF, OIF, and OND veterans like Jamie be screened for possible TBI. Those who screen positive must be offered specialized evaluation and treatment. The VA's 2016 clear general treatment recommendations meet the common-sense test. Treatment shouldn't depend on how long ago the injury occurred, what the symptoms relate to, or what caused them. More and more mild TBIs among active duty servicemen and women are being diagnosed, just as civilian concussion numbers have increased.

The DVBIC reports that from 2000 to 2011, the annual incidence of TBI climbed from 400 per 100,000 to 1,400 per 100,000. The numbers are also climbing as the VA evaluates the backlog of members who may have had a TBI and are transitioning from the military to VA health-care systems. For many different reasons, only about 50 percent of eligible veterans use the VA system. In 2016, an accusation that the VA employed unqualified medical specialists to perform about 25,000 veteran evaluations (out of the more than a million evaluations performed on returning veterans) was investigated in Congressional hearings, and the VA acknowledged the problem. Service members were recalled and reexamined by experts in neurology, neurosurgery, physiatry, and psychiatry to rectify this problem.

The Long Haul

The long-term effects of TBI and its related conditions can be far more serious than a clinician may initially predict, especially if left untreated. Studies show that, just as with repetitive sports concussions, multiple concussions sustained on the battlefield or in other military operations can lead to aggressive behaviors, poor impulse control, depression to the point of suicide, and even dementia. Just like athletes, military personnel may be reluctant to report symptoms, as Jamie was. They may be inclined to brush it off because they want to remain with their unit, meet the expectations of peers and superiors, and not jeopardize their careers. If untreated, some symptoms may worsen, and others may emerge. Use of alcohol, tobacco, and nonprescribed drugs or other substances often increases immediately following a mild TBI.

Over the longer term, the possibility of developing a neurodegenerative disease (ND) looms large. The VA estimates that more than 75 percent of US veterans have Alzheimer's disease or another form of dementia, and the number of VA enrollees with Alzheimer's grew 166 percent from 2004 to 2014. In a study of more than 180,000 veterans, neurologist Kristine Yaffe and her colleagues found that those diagnosed with PTSD had twice the risk of dementia in veterans without PTSD. The TBI–PTSD debate has carried over into ND research as well.

Not surprisingly, there are associations between military TBIs and CTE, just as there are for athletes subjected to repetitive concussions. Bennet Omalu (the pathologist who diagnosed CTE in Mike Webster's brain) published a case of CTE in a 27-year-old Iraqi Marine and war veteran who committed suicide after deployments that exposed him to IEDs. The veteran developed cognitive impairments, mood disorders that included PTSD, and a substance use disorder. Boston University pathologist Ann McKee and her colleagues have found CTE in the brains of marines, soldiers, and sailors who served in World War II and the Vietnam, Gulf, Iraq, and Afghanistan wars. More and more veterans, including the former VA secretary Robert McDonald, have pledged to donate their brains for research.

Other High-Risk Occupations

Like military personnel, police and other law enforcement personnel, correction officers, emergency medical workers, and firefighters are at high risk for TBIs, and especially concussions. Falls, vehicle crashes, and blows to the head most commonly injure people in these high-risk occupations. Firefighters on ladders and unstable surfaces near exploding structures clearly work in harm's way. Assaults and high-speed chases threaten police officers.

The top most dangerous jobs, according to the Bureau of Labor Statistics, are logging, fishing, aircraft piloting, roofing, trash and recycling collecting, iron and steel work, truck and sales driving, farming and ranching, construction, and grounds and maintenance work. Severe TBIs cause more than half of the recorded deaths in construction, transportation, agriculture, forestry (logging), and fishing industries. The National Institute for Occupational Safety and Health (NIOSH) reports that the construction industry has the highest number of both fatal and nonfatal traumatic brain injuries among US occupations.

Pablo had become an expert at installing windows while balancing on dangerously dangling scaffolding. He understood the risk he took every time he climbed to do his work. But as he approached his sixtieth birthday, he worried that his risk of falling would increase. He also knew that his new employer was less strict about safety issues than his last boss had been. He accepted this trade-off because he thought the wage increase justified the danger. He was working alone when he fell, but his co-workers heard him cry out as he dropped and then landed on concrete.

Upon waking, Pablo's first memory was of the ambulance siren screaming as they sped down the highway. The pains in his head, arm, and chest were excruciating. He thought about his buddy Greg, an electrician who had taken a high-voltage hit and fallen off scaffolding several years before, becoming permanently disabled. The emergency room doctor recorded multiple rib fractures, a right wrist fracture, and a Glasgow Coma Scale (GCS) of 15. The CT scan the doctor ordered did not show any bleeding in the brain, although there was a small skull fracture.

At construction sites, falls like Pablo's are the most common cause of a TBI. Fall rates are highest among the youngest (least experienced) and oldest workers, and workers 65 years and older have the highest TBI fatality rate of all age groups. As the workforce ages, so do injuries to older workers, often from falls. Injurious falls can happen even in office environments, on wet or uneven surfaces, or tripping over objects that are out of place. Occupational TBI death rates have declined in the United States, but nonfatal work-related rates have substantially increased, especially for fall-related injuries. One study found occupational fatality rates fifteen times higher for men, because most of the high-risk occupations are male-dominated.

Electricians risk high-voltage injuries that include burns, nerve damage, or cardiac arrest and its catastrophic consequences. However, a concussion or more severe TBI can occur with a fall off a ladder, or as in Pablo's friend Greg's case, when an electrical surge enters the body. What is referred to as a diffuse electrical injury is a rare and challenging diagnosis that occurs with lower-voltage injuries (1,000 volts or less). These patients may have symptoms such as pain in the hand or arm, explained by the path of the electrical current. But the reason they are called diffuse injuries is that other symptoms—headaches, dizziness, fatigue, memory problems, and symptoms that may typically follow concussions—may not be clearly connected to the path of the current through the body into the brain. There may be a delay (days or weeks) before symptoms emerge, and physical signs or neuroimaging findings may not confirm the diagnosis. Following a thorough evaluation for other causes of the symptoms, treatment approaches like those for other patients with a history of concussion or mild TBI work well.

Technical theater workers, such as lighting technicians or stage managers, are also at high risk for a TBI. These workers do multiple activities similar to the tasks of construction workers or electricians. In one study, two-thirds of theater workers had experienced a head injury. About 40 percent reported having had five or more head injuries. More than half of the workers did not report the injury despite post-concussion symptoms. Low lighting conditions, complex and unwieldy backstage equipment, and physical contact during activities such as stage combat all contribute to the risk. Stunt doubles and actors who do their own stunts, like Jackie Chan, also suffer concussions.

The Jockeys

Any discussion of occupational injuries must include jockeys, because one of the most hazardous occupations is riding racehorses. Jockeys are among the most fit of athletes, yet their fitness does not necessarily protect them. Racehorses weigh more than a ton and on average travel at speeds around forty miles per hour. Jockeys are injured most often by a fall from a horse or falling when a horse tumbles or collapses. Some jockeys are trampled or crushed by a fallen horse after they fall. Fractures below the neck are the most common injuries, but injuries to the head, face, and neck are the next most common. Within this second list are concussion and more severe TBIs along with spinal cord injury with paralysis.

Physiatrist Joel Press and colleagues at the Rehabilitation Institute of Chicago and Kaiser Permanente published results of a national survey of 706 jockeys in the 1990s. Over the course of four months, these jockeys suffered more than 1,700 injuries. Jockeys reported an average of three injuries per year. Concussions occurred in 13 percent of the jockeys surveyed. That rate, as the authors pointed out, is much higher than the rate for football or boxing. More recently, Peta Hitchens, a University of California, Davis researcher, and her colleagues reported that 180 California jockeys fell 505 times and 269 suffered injuries during a five-year period from 2007 to 2011. Sixty-one percent fell more than once during that period. The most common reason for jockey falls was catastrophic injury or death of a horse, and 60 percent of the time this also means serious or catastrophic injuries for the jockey.

Although jockey injury rates overall have declined since the 1980s due to increased safety measures, including improved helmets, they remain alarming. In *Seabiscuit: An American Legend,* Laura Hillenbrand captured what jockeys do with fear given these grim statistics: "jockeys never, ever spoke about danger, pain, or fear, even among themselves. In conversation they papered over the grim realities of their jobs with cheery euphemisms. Hideous wrecks were referred to as 'spills'; jockeys hurled into the ground were 'unseated.' In their autobiographies, they recounted great races in intimate detail, but falls and injuries were glossed over with the most perfunctory language. Even in the grip of agonizing pain or complete debilitation, most jockeys clung to their illusion of invulnerability." Jockeys make up a relatively small group of people, but a group we must not forget in discussions of concussions and dangerous occupations.

Care and Outcomes of Injured Workers

Workplace injury research suggests that people injured at work typically have a greater risk of delayed return to work and other poor outcomes compared to those not injured at work. Unfortunately, there are few well-designed studies of workers with concussion or mild TBI. Neuropsychologist Douglas Terry and his Harvard colleagues studied workers and nonworkers with a history of a mild TBI using a case-control method (with a case group and a control group). The worker group consisted of more men who had lower education levels and fewer holding managerial or professional jobs, but the group outcomes were similar. Approximately 40 percent of those in both groups fully returned to work or were approved to return to work between six and seven months from injury. Unfortunately, almost the same percentage had not returned to work in that time frame. The two groups did not differ in terms of risk factors associated with prolonged absence from work and were similar in that post-concussion symptoms predicted no return to work.

Workers who experience concussions may suffer persistent post-concussion symptoms for months. The symptoms may interfere with work and work productivity. New Zealand researcher Alice Theadom and colleagues found that at four years after a mild TBI, 17 percent of workers had exited the workforce (other than for retirement or educational reasons) or were working reduced hours compared with their schedules before the injury. In addition, close to 16 percent reported that the injury limited them at work. Those who had the symptom "taking longer to think" at one month experienced the most productivity loss after four years. These researchers concluded that health-care professionals must identify cognitive problems and implement interventions to address them immediately after an injury.

These studies do not answer questions about effective interventions to return people to work after these injuries. Comprehensive and coordinated approaches to medical care and rehabilitation may produce much better statistics for injured workers who need comprehensive, multifaceted treatment programs. Northern California clinical neuropsychologist Ernest Bryant, who has decades of experience evaluating injured workers and other patients with TBIs, put it this way: "Work place mild traumatic brain injuries should be taken very seriously. They may be mild in degree but their impact on recovery and return to work can be profound. Patients can develop chronic, disabling cognitive and psychiatric conditions, and substance abuse. There can be many psychological and social stressors, and litigation adds stress as well. Assessments and subsequent treatments should be provided in a coordinated and comprehensive fashion, preferably in a brain injury rehabilitation program model."

Pablo and Jamie

Even after treatment for benign paroxysmal positional vertigo (BPPV), neck pain and headaches, and cognitive problems, Pablo's injury threatened his ability to work in the six months following his injury (see Chapter 3). A repeat neuropsychological evaluation at that time showed significant improvements in his thinking and memory, although he still had mild problems with attention, concentration, and short-term memory. A functional capacity evaluation, paid for through workers' compensation, showed Pablo quite capable of returning to work in a construction or construction-related industry. These evaluations suggested that he was able to do some work, just not the kind of work he had done before on scaffolding. His neuropsychologist suggested that the accommodations at work include providing him with written in addition to verbal instructions for new skill acquisition.

Pablo participated in vocational counseling and supported employment programs at a home improvement store. He stocked items and helped people find what they needed. Eventually, he was able to serve as a contractor's resource in the store's building supply area. He never went up on scaffolding or ladders over four feet again. Pablo worked hard and delighted in his new job. Two years after his injury, Pablo was promoted to assistant store manager. His concussion symptoms resolved.

The army sent Jamie home from the battlefield for comprehensive treatment and rehabilitation under the care of a VA physiatrist. A psychiatrist and a psychologist evaluated and treated Jamie for PTSD and depression. He began taking an antidepressant, and his symptoms gradually improved. Jamie did not return to military duty. His VA physiatrist and psychiatrist determined he had a service-related disability. He continued to attend speech therapy for his cognitive impairments. He was able to live alone with support from his family, and he also found a supportive community at his local church. His VA social worker encouraged him to volunteer at a local food kitchen for the homeless. He felt grateful that his life had new meaning and purpose, and his service animal became his constant companion. He continued to receive medical care at a local VA clinic.

Final Words

The war theater and certain workplaces carry inherent risks for concussion and more severe TBIs. Every supervisor in the civilian or military setting, and every employee or person in military service, must play a part to prevent TBIs. Falling off scaffolding as Pablo did should never happen. In the world of work, federal standards are set by the US Department of Labor's Occupational Safety and Health Administration (OSHA). OSHA provides free and confidential consultation for workers and employers. These services can identify workplace hazards, evaluate compliance with standards, and help establish safety and health programs. Businesses with ten or fewer employees, and some religious organizations and other entities, are exempt from OSHA requirements for inspections and injury or incident reporting. The Board of Certified Safety Professionals (BCSP) and NIOSH partner to protect the safety and health of workers and provide education and certification programs and other services.

Of course, prevention is not always possible, which is why we must have the resources to treat injured soldiers and workers. My colleague Michael Choo, emergency medicine physician and chief medical officer of Paradigm, emphasized the importance of engaging brain injury experts and coordination of care for injured workers with concussions and more severe injuries: "When it comes to TBI, our expectations are currently set too low for injured workers and veterans. We cannot and must not capitulate to the status quo. Rather we must strive to achieve the best functional outcomes possible with systematic care management and the best brain injury experts. Exponential growth in our knowledge about TBI through research will most certainly improve brain recovery and brain health in the future."

The Department of Defense and the VA require steady, comprehensive funding for human resources and technologies to diagnose and treat the thousands of people who have served our nation. So, too, must the workers' compensation industry rise to meet the challenge of diagnosing and treating workers with brain injuries, and be properly funded to do so.

Conclusion

W E ARE FINALLY coming to our senses about concussion, which scientists and physicians have for centuries called *commotio cerebri* (shaken brain), an injury to the brain that was often not considered serious or permanent. Researchers have begun to unveil the brain's mysteries, along with the mystery of what happens when the brain is shaken. It takes a long time for the brain to mature, with a lot of construction and remodeling taking place in the months before birth and for decades after birth. Early in life, and then again late in life, our brains are most vulnerable to injury. Concussions can disrupt that maturation process.

Care and Treatment

Diagnosing a concussion is a multifaceted endeavor because a concussion disorders the brain in complex ways. Because we lack precise clinical tools and measures, predicting outcomes with certainty is difficult. However, a physician trained and experienced in brain injury medicine and concussion, who understands the consequences of physical and psychological trauma to the brain, can make medically-based decisions that do improve outcomes. We also need a team of other providers—neuropsychologists, neuro-ophthalmologists, neuro-optometrists, and physical, occupational, and speech therapists—to meet the needs of people with concussions.

Although we have no magic pill and no crystal ball, there are symptomatic treatments, pertinent education and advice, rehabilitation interventions, and self-management strategies for managing a concussion's aftermath. Specific physical, psychological, and cognitive therapies can speed recovery, as can targeted medications. We can be cautiously optimistic about outcomes for people who have had only one concussion. Most concussion patients are eventually able to return to school, work, play, or redeployment after a single injury.

One concussion, however, can increase the risk of additional concussions. People are especially vulnerable to a second concussion if it occurs before a full recovery from the first. Symptom reports are not the best measure of recovery, but in the absence of biomarkers, they are all we have to rely on. This means that we must take a conservative approach—adding more time after symptom resolution—before risking another injury. Recurrent concussions, such as those that occur in all collision or combat sports, are more likely than a single concussion to result in prolonged or incomplete recoveries. Devastating diseases such as chronic traumatic encephalopathy (CTE) are increasingly linked to a history of multiple concussions in susceptible people.

At-Risk Groups

Exercise benefits the brain and body, and there are lots of ways to participate in sports and recreation without risking a concussion.

We need to encourage our children and youth to participate in physical activities (including team sports) with the lowest risks of concussion. Unfortunately, societies that revere competitive sports push many young athletes in ways that lead to multiple concussions, with retirement from a sport occurring only after far too much damage has already been done, damage that affects a young person's future off the field as well as on it.

In the United States, falls cause the largest number of brain injuries, especially for the very young and those over 65. Pediatric abusive head trauma (AHT) and intimate partner violence (IPV) affect a frequently undiagnosed and untreated population of concussion patients. Women are more likely than men to suffer concussions and other injuries from IPV, often repetitive injuries accompanied by psychic trauma that interacts with and exacerbates the physical trauma. Prisoners, homeless people, and others who live at the margins of society face high risks of injuries that include concussions, and disadvantaged populations often have scant or no access to resources for evaluation and treatment.

Concussions also take a major toll on brain functioning in workplaces and on the battlefield. Military personnel in combat zones experience high rates of brain injury as well as mental health disorders, including post-traumatic stress disorder (PTSD), depression, and substance use disorder.

Everyone who experiences a concussion deserves expert care.

Personal, Institutional, and Global Responsibilities

In this book, I offer some personal prevention strategies. Young athletes and their parents, and coaches and other school professionals, must learn what they can about concussion—the science, the symptoms, and the recommendations for equipment, safe play, removal from and return to play, and retirement from playing a sport. Parents, grandparents, and caregivers can learn about nursery and other children's products and safety strategies in the home and car and on playgrounds. Workers must report unsafe conditions to their supervisors, and company leaders and managers need to take responsibility for keeping their employees safe. The elderly and people with disabilities, along with their families and supporters, need to adopt fall prevention strategies. Victims can seek help for IPV and parents can learn to manage frustrations that lead to pediatric AHT.

Concussion is not just a personal or a family problem, however. It is a public health problem that must be addressed through national and international efforts. Our global community needs the courage to confront the nexus of competition, money, politics, and culture that drives the sports–industrial complex. Those who think the entire concussion problem has been overblown amplify their views on social media and disseminate harmful misinformation. Denial of the problem overlaps with conflicts of interest, both institutional and individual, that interfere with research, the development of guidelines, and efforts to prevent concussions and their consequences.

We need to effectively educate athletes and those who are responsible for protecting them from injury with evidence-based information and guidance. We must not tell them to "just shake it off," and we must find more effective educational strategies. We must do more research to establish what other interventions, such as changing play rules, can lower the risk of injury. Redesigning athletic equipment can mitigate injuries. However, some equipment may actually heighten the risks of concussion or more severe brain injury, giving athletes a false sense of security and encouraging them to play more aggressively. Much more research is needed in all these areas.

We must reduce the number and severity of falls in the very young, the elderly, and people with disabilities; work to eliminate IPV and pediatric AHT; decrease the number and severity of assaults among incarcerated and homeless populations, and improve traffic and transportation safety. Workplaces need to develop better prevention plans, enforce regulations, educate managers and workers about risks, and ensure full compliance. It is clearly time to develop clinical guidelines for workplace brain injuries and risk-reduction strategies for high-risk occupations. Military personnel and veterans need access to specialized and comprehensive care after brain injuries. Rehabilitation services remain incommensurate with the number of people affected by our ongoing wars. Funding for veterans' clinical care and research has always been highly subject to the prevailing political winds and needs to be ensured.

Achieving these goals will require multipronged and far-reaching national and international efforts that combine multifaceted research programs, public policy reforms, public health programs, education, and clinical training programs. Moves in all these directions could improve the health and quality of life of millions of people in the United States and worldwide. The time is now.

NOTES ON THE TEXT

Preface

Physiatrists Sheldon Berrol, Nathan Cope, Lawrence Horn, Nathaniel Mayer, and Henry Stonnington were early pioneers of brain injury rehabilitation in the 1970s and 1980s, long before the American Board of Medical Specialties officially declared brain injury medicine (BIM) a medical specialty (in 2011). Neurologists Michael Alexander, Sanford Auerbach, and Douglas Katz led the way in neurology and Thomas McAllister, Gregory O'Shanick, and Jonathan Silver played a similar role in psychiatry. Physiatrists, neurologists, and psychiatrists can now seek board certification in this new medical specialty.

An account of the early period of brain injury medicine can be found in D. N. Cope, M. E. Sandel, et al. 2013. "Dr. Sheldon Berrol: Champion of Brain Injury Rehabilitation and Disability Rights," *PM&R* 5(11):907–914.

1 What Happens to the Brain?

In the 1990s, I participated in early research at the University of Pennsylvania, using various advanced neuroimaging techniques to study patients with chronic symptoms after concussion. These techniques, namely magnetic resonance spectroscopy (MRS), positron emission tomography (PET), and single photon emission tomography (SPECT), suggested that the brains of people with concussion show subtle abnormalities and that the hippocampus and the corpus callosum might be particularly vulnerable. See these sources for additional information.

a) K. M. Cecil, E. C. Hills, M. E. Sandel, et al. 1998. "Proton Magnetic Resonance Spectroscopy for Detection of Axonal Injury in the Splenium of the Corpus Callosum of Brain-Injured Patients." *Journal of Neurosurgery* 88(5):795–801.

b) E. M. Umile, R. C. Plotkin, and M. E. Sandel. 1998. "Functional Assessment of Mild Traumatic Brain Injury Using SPECT and Neuropsychological Testing." *Brain Injury* 12(7):577–594.

c) E. M. Umile, M. E. Sandel, A. Alavi, et al. 2002. "Dynamic Imaging in Mild Traumatic Brain Injury: Support for the Theory of Medial Temporal Vulnerability." *Archives of Physical Medicine and Rehabilitation* 83(11):1506–1513.

The Banyan Biomarker website contains additional information about the company's progress in biomarker research: https://www.banyanbio .com/.

2   The Search for a Diagnosis

The following experts provided information in personal communications: Ernest Bryant, PhD, March 15, 2019; Stephen Casper, PhD, September 16, 2018; Seth Fischer, MD, April 25 and 27, 2017; Mel Glenn, MD, November 5, 2018; Steven Moskowitz, MD, December 8, 2018.

Neurologist Henry Miller's biases are very evident in these quotes: "Amongst the predisposing factors encountered in certain cases was below-average intelligence. A past history of evident emotional instability, invalidism, hypochondriasis, or prolonged incapacity after previous minor injuries . . . a shiftless work record . . . and menopausal nervous symptoms, coincident hypertension, and arteriosclerosis" were other factors he cited.

Miller labeled behaviors such as "dramatization of symptoms," a patient "slumping forward with head in hands during the consultation, requesting a glass of water." And he went on in this vein: "I had long regarded this last as a pathognomonic [specific for the disease itself] sign of accident neurosis, but I understand that it is often seen in women requesting termination of pregnancy on psychiatric grounds."

The authors of the latest International Consensus Statement on concussion in sport continue to use the term *functional,* in contrast to *structural,* to describe concussion. They then hedge a bit by saying that sports-related concussion "may result in neuropathological changes, but the acute clinical signs and symptoms largely reflect a functional disturbance rather than a structural injury and, as such, no abnormality is seen on standard structural neuroimaging studies." With advanced neuroimaging, we see more and more evidence of structural injury to the brain after concussion or even "subconcussion" (brain trauma without symptoms or signs), a term used as early as the 1940s.

I came to the unfortunate realization over many decades that PCS remains a challenging and complex condition that is not always taken seriously by the medical profession. This sentence in an article I wrote in the 1990s still rings true: "Since most patients are discharged from an emergency room with a minor brain injury without any preparation or warning as to what to expect, the subsequent occurrence of postconcussional symptoms and cognitive deficits may be extremely distressing and limiting and may lead to the fear of permanent impairment or disability." (A. S. Zwil, M. E. Sandel, and E. Kim. 1993. "Organic and Psychological Sequelae of Traumatic Brain Injury: The Postconcussional Syndrome in Clinical Practice." *New Directions in Mental Health Services* 57:109–115).

Strictly speaking, the term PCS is a misnomer because PCS is not a syndrome. A syndrome is a group of symptoms and signs in a pattern that occurs consistently in patients with a particular disorder. This lack of "fit" has led some experts to argue that the best terms for the condition are post-concussive disorder or post-concussional disorder. In fact, there has not been agreement among professional organizations (such as the World Health Organization, the American Psychiatric Association, and the American Congress of Rehabilitation Medicine) about the definitions of the symptomatic conditions people experience after a concussion.

Santa Clara Valley Medical Center, along with other Traumatic Brain Injury Model Systems Programs, funded by the National Institute on Disability and Rehabilitation Research, coordinates the Center for Outcomes Research in Brain Injury. This site has information about various testing instruments used by neuropsychologists and other rehabilitation professionals: http://www.tbims.org/.

3 Concussion Care

The following experts provided information in personal communications: David Cifu, MD, December 19, 2019; Mel Glenn, MD, January 2, 2019; Nathan Zasler, MD, March 24, 2019.

These three concussion / mild TBI websites provide guidelines for practitioners as well as educational materials for the public:

a) CDC Pediatric Mild TBI Guideline: https://www.cdc.gov/traumatic braininjury/PediatricmTBIGuideline.html.
b) CDC Adult mild TBI Guideline: https://www.cdc.gov/traumatic braininjury/mtbi_guideline.html.
c) Ontario Neurotrauma Foundation Guidelines: http://onf.org/our -programs/acquired-brain-injury/concussion-mild-tbi.

The American Academy of Physical Medicine and Rehabilitation lists physiatrists with subspecialty board certification in brain injury medicine, sports medicine, and pain medicine: https://members.aapmr.org/AAPMR /AAPMR_FINDER.aspx.

The Concussion Legacy Foundation provides helpful tips and a search tool for choosing a sports concussion clinic: https://concussionfoundation .org/concussion-resources/concussion-clinics/tips-choosing-concussion -clinic.

4 Long-Term Risks

On the subject of *League of Denial* (book and film), see:

a) M. Fainaru-Wada and S. Fainaru. 2013. *League of Denial: The NFL, Concussions and the Battle for the Truth.* New York: Crown Publishing.
b) Public Broadcasting Service (PBS). 2013. "League of Denial: The NFL's Concussion Crisis." *Frontline.* https://www.pbs.org/wgbh/pages/frontline/oral-history/league-of-denial.

Bennet Omalu's life and work are discussed or represented in these sources:

a) J. M. Laskas. 2015. *Concussion.* New York: Random House.
b) *Concussion,* released in 2015 by Warner Brothers / Sony Pictures.
d) J. M. Laskas. 2009. "Bennet Omalu, Concussions, and the NFL: How One Doctor Changed Football Forever." *GQ,* September 14.
e) B. Omalu and W. Smith. 2017. *Truth Doesn't Have a Side: My Alarming Discovery About the Danger of Contact Sports.* New York: Harper Collins.

NHL enforcer Derek Boogaard's story can be found in J. Branch, "'I Don't Want People to Forget Him': The NFL Has Been Consumed by the Concussion Issue. Why Hasn't the N.H.L.?" *New York Times,* June 2, 2019.

5 Exercising Sensibly

The US Consumer Product Safety Commission's helmet advice is found here: https://www.cpsc.gov/safety-education/safety-guides/sports-fitness-and-recreation-bicycles/which-helmet-which-activity.

See the National Electronic Injury Surveillance System on sports-related injuries: https://www.cpsc.gov/Research—Statistics/NEISS-Injury-Data/.

The National Household Travel Survey and associated data is found here: https://nhts.ornl.gov/.

The CDC information about playground injuries is found here: https://www.cdc.gov/safechild/playground/.

6 Game Changers

The CDC has many educational resources for athletes, parents, coaches, and school and healthcare professionals: https://www.cdc.gov/HEADSUP/.

7 Money Talks

This is a brief but relevant article on conflicts of interest in medicine: C. C. Muth. 2017. "Conflicts of Interest in Medicine." *JAMA* 317(17):1812. doi:10.1001/jama; https://jamanetwork.com/journals/jama/fullarticle/2623608.

8 Close to Home

The following experts provided information in personal communications: Maya Evans, MD, November 29, 2018; Brigid McCaw, MD, November 26, 2018.

An excellent resource on nursery safety is found here: https://www.nationwidechildrens.org/research/areas-of-research/center-for-injury-research-and-policy/injury-topics/home-safety/nursery-safety.

Government websites with resources on children's safety and health:

a) Nursery products, Consumer Product Safety Commission (CPSC): https://www.cpsc.gov/safety-education/safety-guides/kids-and-babies/safe-nursery.

b) Product instability–related injuries: A. Suchy, "Product Instability or Tip-Over Injuries and Fatalities Associated with Televisions, Furniture and Appliances: 2018 Report." https://www.cpsc.gov/content/product-instability-or-tip-over-injuries-and-fatalities-associated-with-televisions-1.

c) The National Child Abuse and Neglect Data System (NCANDS). Children's Bureau, Health and Human Services: https://www.acf.hhs.gov/cb/research-data-technology/reporting-systems/ncands.

d) Centers for Disease Control and Prevention (CDC), Pediatric AHT: S. E. Parks, J. L. Annest, and H. A. Hill. 2012. "Pediatric Abusive Head Trauma: Recommended Definitions for Public Health Surveillance and Research." https://www.cdc.gov/violenceprevention/pdf/pedhead trauma-a.pdf.

e) National Institute of Child Health and Development's Safe to Sleep Campaign: https://safetosleep.nichd.nih.gov/activities/campaign.

These sites address the health and safety of elders:

a) US Department of Justice, support for victims and families: https://www .justice.gov/elderjustice/support/faq.html#what-is-elder-abuse.

b) National Center on Elder Abuse (NCEA), Administration on Aging. Statistic / data: http://ncea.acl.gov/Library/Data/index.aspx.

c) CDC: http://www.cdc.gov/violenceprevention/elderabuse/index.html.

d) World Elder Abuse Awareness Day: https://ncea.acl.gov/.

e) World Health Organization (WHO). "Elder abuse." Updated 8 June 2018. https://www.who.int/news-room/fact-sheets/detail/elder-abuse.

f) Falls prevention for older adults: J. A. Stevens and E. R. Burns. "A CDC Compendium of Effective Fall Interventions: What Works for Community-Dwelling Older Adults." 3rd ed. Atlanta, GA: CDC, National Center for Injury Prevention and Control, 2015. https://www .cdc.gov/homeandrecreationalsafety/pdf/falls/cdc_falls_compendium -2015-a.pdf.

9 War and Work

Individuals providing personal communications: Ernest Bryant, PhD, March 15, 2019; Stephen Casper, PhD, September 16, 2018; Michael Choo, MD, March 14, 2019; David Cifu, MD, August 18, 2018.

Charles Hoge's research stirred controversy within the research community about whether symptoms and outcomes of military concussions and blast injuries were due to PTSD or brain injury. See these letters to the editor of the *New England Journal of Medicine:* "Mild Traumatic Brain Injury in U.S. Soldiers Returning from Iraq," *New England Journal of Medicine* 358: 20, and "Care of War Veterans with Traumatic Brain Injury," *New England Journal of Medicine* 361: 536–538.

Government and other websites:

a) Department of Veterans Affairs. 2017. "Traumatic Brain Injury and PTSD: Focus on Veterans - PTSD: National Center for PTSD": https://www.ptsd.va.gov/professional/co-occurring/traumatic-brain -injury-ptsd.asp.

b) Department of Veterans Affairs, and Department of Defense. 2016. "VA / DoD Clinical Practice Guideline for the Management of Concussion—Mild Traumatic Brain Injury," February: 1–133. https://www.healthquality.va.gov/guidelines/Rehab/mtbi/.

c) US Department of Defense—Suicide Prevention: https://dod.defense .gov/News/Special-Reports/0915_suicideprevention/.

d) National Institute for Occupational Health and Safety: https://www .cdc.gov/niosh/index.htm.

e) US Department of Labor–Workers Compensation: https://www.dol .gov/owcp/.

Conclusion

In 2011, the National Institutes of Health and the European Commission organized a workshop that led to important international efforts. That same year, I had the opportunity to join an international panel on TBI research at the meeting of the Annual Neurotrauma National Symposium in Las Vegas that was related to these efforts. Subsequently, I participated in the Traumatic Brain Injury Common Data Elements Project (Rehabilitation Subgroup) sponsored by the National Institute of Neurological Disorders and Stroke and other federal agencies: https://www.commondataelements .ninds.nih.gov/TBI.aspx#tab=Data_Standards.

REFERENCES

Preface

Anderson, V., C. Godfrey, J. V. Rosenfeld, et al. 2012. "Predictors of Cognitive Function and Recovery 10 Years after Traumatic Brain Injury in Young Children." *Pediatrics* 129(2):e254–261.

Basen, R. 2017. "Brain Injuries in Sport Are Real Public Health Problem, Senators Told." *MedPage Today,* May 19. https://www.medpagetoday .com/sportsmedicine/generalsportsmedicine/65447.

BlueCross / BlueShield. 2016. "The Health of America Report: The Steep Rise in Concussion Diagnosis in the U.S." https://www.bcbs.com /the-health-of-america/reports/the-steep-rise-concussion-diagnoses -the-us.

Buck, P. W., R. G. Laster, J. S. Sagrati, et al. 2012. "Working with Mild Traumatic Brain Injury: Voices from the Field." *Rehabilitation Research and Practice* 2012:1–6. See p. 3.

Centers for Disease Control and Prevention. 2015. *Report to Congress on Traumatic Brain Injury in the United States: Epidemiology and Rehabilitation.*

National Center for Injury Prevention and Control, Division of Unintentional Injury Prevention, CDC, Atlanta, GA. http://www.cdc.gov/traumaticbraininjury/pdf/TBI_Report_to_Congress_Epi_and_Rehab-a.pdf.

Defense and Veterans Brain Injury Center. 2018. "DoD Worldwide Numbers for TBI." http://dvbic.dcoe.mil/dod-worldwide-numbers-tbi.

DePadilla L., G. F. Miller, S. E. Jones, et al. 2018. "Self-Reported Concussions from Playing a Sport or Being Physically Active among High School Students—United States, 2017." *Morbidity and Mortality Weekly Report* 67(24):682–685.

Eisenberg, M. A., W. P. Meehan, and R. Mannix. 2014. "Duration and Course of Post-Concussive Symptoms." *Pediatrics* 133(6):999–1006.

Gaw, C. E., and M. R. Zonfrillo. 2016. "Emergency Department Visits for Head Trauma in the United States." *BMC Emergency Medicine* 16:5.

Hiploylee, C., P. A. Dufort, H. S. Davis, et al. 2017. "Longitudinal Study of Postconcussive Syndrome: Not Everyone Recovers." *Journal of Neurotrauma* 34:1511–1523.

Hippocrates. 1928. *On Wounds in the Head.* Trans. E. T. Withington. Hippocrates, vol. 3. Loeb Classical Library 149. Cambridge, MA: Harvard University Press.

"How Knowledgeable Are Americans about Concussions? Assessing and Recalibrating the Public's Knowledge." 2015. University of Pittsburgh Medical Center, September 30. Full report of Harris poll available through http://rethinkconcussions.upmc.com/2015/09/concussion-survey/.

McMahon, P., A. Hricik, J. K. Yue, et al. 2014. "Symptomatology and Functional Outcome in Mild Traumatic Brain Injury: Results from the Prospective TRACK-TBI Study." *Journal of Neurotrauma* 31:26–33.

"Poll: Nearly 1 in 4 Americans Report Having a Concussion." 2016. NPR, *All Things Considered,* May 31. http://www.npr.org/sections/health-shots/2016/05/31/479750268/poll-nearly-1-in-4-americans-report-having-had-a-concussion.

Sarmiento, K., K. E. Thomas, J. Daugherty, et al. 2019. "Emergency Department Visits for Sports- and Recreation-Related Traumatic Brain Injuries among Children—United States, 2010–2016." *Morbidity and Mortality Weekly Report* 68(10):237–242.

Seabury, S. A., E. Gaudette, and E. P. Goldman. 2018. "Assessment of Follow-up Care after Emergency Department Presentation for Mild Traumatic Brain Injury." *JAMA Network Open* 1(1):e180210.

Tator, C. H., H. S. Davis, P. A. Dufort, et al. 2016. "Postconcussion Syndrome: Demographics and Predictors in 221 Patients." *Journal of Neurosurgery* 125(5):1206–1216.

Theadom, A., V. Parag, T. Dowell, et al. 2014. "Persistent Problems 1 Year after Mild Traumatic Brain Injury: A Longitudinal Population Study in New Zealand." *British Journal of General Practice* 66(642):e16–e23.

Theadom, A., N. Starkey, S. Barker-Collo, et al. 2018. "Population-Based Cohort Study of the Impacts of Mild Traumatic Brain Injury in Adults Four Years Post-Injury." *PLoS One* 13(1):e0191655.

Valera, E. M., A. Cao, O. Pasternak, et al. 2019. "White Matter Correlates of Mild Traumatic Brain Injury in Women Subjected to Intimate-Partner Violence: A Preliminary Study." *Journal of Neurotrauma* 36(5):661–668.

Veliz, P., S. E. McCabe, J. T. Eckner, et al. 2017. "Research Letter: Prevalence of Concussion among US Adolescents and Correlated Factors." *JAMA* 318:1180–1182.

World Health Organization. n.d. ICD-10 Codes (concussion—S06.0). https://icd.who.int/browse10/2016/en#/S06.0. Accessed September 10, 2019.

Chapter 1 ▪ What Happens to the Brain?

Adams, J. H., D. Doyle, I. Ford, et al. 1989. "Diffuse Axonal Injury in Head Injury: Definition, Diagnosis, and Grading." *Histopathology* 15(1):49–59.

Adams, J. H., D. I. Graham, L. S. Murray, et al. 1982. "Diffuse Axonal Injury Due to Nonmissile Head Injury in Humans: An Analysis of 45 Cases." *Annuals of Neurology* 12:557–563.

Alhilali, L. M., K. Yaeger, M. Collins, et al. 2014. "Detection of Central White Matter Injury Underlying Vestibulopathy after Mild Traumatic Brain Injury." *Radiology* 272(1):224–232.

Asken, B. M., S. T. DeKosky, J. R. Clugston, et al. 2018. "Diffusion Tensor Imaging (DTI) Findings in Adult Civilian, Military, and Sport-Related Mild Traumatic Brain Injury (mTBI): A Systematic Critical Review." *Brain Imaging and Behavior* 12:585–612.

Barkhoudarian, G., D. A. Hovda, and C. C. Giza. 2011. "The Molecular Pathophysiology of Concussive Brain Injury." *Clinics in Sports Medicine* 30(1):33–48.

Barth, J. T., J. R. Freeman, D. K. Broshek, et al. 2001. "Acceleration-Deceleration Sport-Related Concussion: The Gravity of It All." *Journal of Athletic Training* 36(3):253–256.

Bigler, E. D., T. J. Abildskov, N. J. Goodrich-Hunsaker, et al. 2016. "Structural Neuroimaging Findings in Mild Traumatic Brain Injury." *Sports Medicine and Arthroscopy Review* 24(3):e42–52.

Burda, J. E., A. M. Bernstein, and M. V. Sofroniew. 2016. "Astrocyte Roles in Traumatic Brain Injury." *Experimental Neurology* 275: 305–315.

Buttram, S. D. W., P. Garcia-Filion, J. Miller, et al. 2015. "Computed Tomography vs Magnetic Resonance Imaging for Identifying Acute Lesions in Pediatric Traumatic Brain Injury." *Hospital Pediatrics* 5(2): 79–84.

Carroll, J. A., B. Race, K. Williams, et al. 2018. "Microglia Are Critical in Host Defense against Prion Disease." *Journal of Virology* 92(15): e00549-18.

Churchill, N. W., M. G. Hutchison, A. P. de Battista, et al. 2017. "Structural, Functional, and Metabolic Brain Markers Differentiate Collision versus Contact and Non-Contact Athletes." *Frontiers in Neurology* 8:390.

Churchill, N. W., M. C. Hutchinson, D. Richards, et al. 2017. "Neuroimaging of Sport Concussion: Persistent Alterations of Brain Structure and Function at Medical Clearance." *Nature: Scientific Reports* 7:8297.

Courville, C. B. 1953. *Commotio Cerebri: Cerebral Concussion and the Postconcussion Syndrome in Their Medical and Legal Aspects.* Los Angeles: San Lucas Press.

Davenport, E. M., C. T. Whitlow, and J. E. Urban. 2014. "Abnormal White Matter Integrity Related to Head Injury Exposure in a Season of High School Varsity Football." *Journal of Neurotrauma* 31:1617–1624.

Dean, P. J. A., J. R. Sato, G. Vieira, et al. 2015. "Long-Term Structural Changes after MTBI and Their Relation to Post-Concussion Symptoms." *Brain Injury* 29(10):1211–1218.

Dennis, E. L., M. U. Ellis, S. D. Marion, et al. 2015. "Callosal Function in Pediatric Traumatic Brain Injury Linked to Disrupted White Matter Integrity." *Journal of Neuroscience* 35(28):10202–10211.

De Simoni, S., P. J. Grover, P. O. Jenkins, et al. 2017. "Disconnection between the Default Mode Network and Medial Temporal Lobes in Post-Traumatic Amnesia." *Brain* 139:3137–3150.

Eierud, C., R. C. Craddock, S. Fletcher, et al. 2014. "Neuroimaging after Mild Traumatic Brain Injury: Review and Meta-Analysis." *Neuro-Image* 4:283–294.

Faden, A. I., J. Wu, B. A. Stoica, et al. 2016. "Progressive Inflammation-Mediated Neurodegeneration after Traumatic Brain or Spinal Cord Injury." *British Journal of Pharmacology* 173(4):681–691.

Fagerholm, E. D., P. J. Hellyer, G. Scott, et al. 2015. "Disconnection of Network Hubs and Cognitive Impairment after Traumatic Brain Injury." *Brain* 138(6):1696–1709.

Farah, G., D. Siwek, and P. Cummings. 2018. "Tau Accumulations in the Brains of Woodpeckers." *PLoS One* 13(2):e091526.

Farkas, O., and J. T. Povlishock. 2007. "Cellular and Subcellular Change Evoked by Diffuse Traumatic Brain Injury: A Complex Web of Change Extending Far beyond Focal Damage." *Progress in Brain Research* 161(6):43–59.

Floyd, C. L., and B. G. Lyeth. 2007. "Astroglia: Important Mediators of Traumatic Brain Injury." *Progress in Brain Research* 161:61–79.

Gawande, A. 2002. *Complications: A Surgeon's Notes on an Imperfect Science.* New York: Picador Books. See p. 7.

Hayes, R., H. Stonnington, B. Lyeth, et al. 1986. "Metabolic and Neurophysiologic Sequelae of Brain Injury: A Cholinergic Hypothesis." *Central Nervous System Trauma* 3(2):163–173.

Hill, C. S., M. P. Coleman, and D. K. Menon. 2016. "Traumatic Axonal Injury: Mechanisms and Translational Opportunities." *Trends in Neurosciences* 39(5):311–324.

Hirad, J. J., K. Bazarian, K. Merchant-Borna, et al. 2019. "A Common Neural Signature of Brain Injury in Concussion and Subconcussion." *Science Advances* 5(8). doi:10.1126/sciadv.aau3460

Huang, Y-L., Y-S. Kuo, Y-C. Tseng, et al. 2015. Susceptibility-Weighted MRI in Mild Traumatic Brain Injury." *Neurology* 84(6):580–585.

Hulkower, M. B., D. B. Poliak, S. B. Rosenbaum, et al. 2013. "A Decade of DTI in Traumatic Brain Injury: 10 Years and 100 Articles Later." *American Journal of Neuroradiology* 11:2064–2074.

Jeter, C. B., G. W. Hergenroeder, M. J. Hylin, et al. 2013. "Biomarkers for the Diagnosis and Prognosis of Mild Traumatic Brain Injury / Concussion." *Journal of Neurotrauma* 30(8):657–670.

Johnson, B., M. Gay, K. Zhang, et al. 2012. "The Use of Magnetic Resonance Spectroscopy in the Subacute Evaluation of Athletes Recovering from Single and Multiple Mild Traumatic Brain Injury." *Journal of Neurotrauma* 29(13):2297–2304.

Katayama, Y., D. P. Becker, T. Tamura, et al. 1990. "Massive Increases in Extracellular Potassium and the Indiscriminate Release of Glutamate Following Concussive Brain Injury." *Journal of Neurosurgery* 73(6): 889–900.

Khong, E., N. Odenwald, E. Hashim, et al. 2016. "Diffusion Tensor Imaging Findings in Post-Concussion Syndrome Patients after Mild Traumatic Brain Injury: A Systematic Review." *Frontiers in Neurology* 7:156.

Lannsjö, M., M. Backheden, U. Johansson, et al. 2013. "Does Head CT Scan Pathology Predict Outcome after Mild Traumatic Brain Injury?" *European Journal of Neurology* 20(1):124–129.

Loane, D. J., and A. Kumar. 2016. "Microglia in the TBI Brain: The Good, the Bad, and the Dysregulated." *Experimental Neurology* 275: 316–327.

May, P. R. A., J. M. Fuster, J. Haber, et al. 1979. "Woodpecker Drilling Behavior: An Endorsement of the Rotational Theory of Impact Brain Injury." *Archives of Neurology* 36(6):370–373.

McGinn, M. J., and J. T. Povlishock. 2015. "Cellular and Molecular Mechanisms of Injury and Spontaneous Recovery." *Handbook of Clinical Neurology* 127:67–87.

Meier, T. B., P. S. F. Bellgowan, R. Singh, et al. "Recovery of Cerebral Blood Flow Following Sports-Related Concussion." *JAMA Neurology* 72(5):530–538.

Misquitta, K., M. Dadar, A. Tarazi, et al. 2018. "The Relationship between Brain Atrophy and Cognitive-Behavioural Symptoms in Retired Canadian Football Players with Multiple Concussions." *Neuroimage: Clinical* 19:551–558.

Moen, K. G., V. Brezova, T. Skandsen, et al. 2014. "Traumatic Axonal Injury: The Prognostic Value of Lesion Load in Corpus Callosum, Brain Stem, and Thalamus in Different Magnetic Resonance Imaging Sequences." *Journal of Neurotrauma* 31(17):1486–1496.

Narayana, P. A., X. Yu, K. M. Hasan, et al. 2015. "Multi-Modal MRI of Mild Traumatic Brain Injury." *Neuroimage: Clinical* 7:87–97.

Niogi, S. N., P. Mukherjee, J. Ghajar, et al. 2008. "Extent of Microstructural White Matter Injury in Postconcussive Syndrome Correlates with Impaired Cognitive Reaction Time: A 3T Diffusion Tensor Imaging Study of Mild Traumatic Brain Injury." *American Journal of Neuroradiology* 29(5):967–973.

Norden, D. M., M. M. Muccigrosso, and J. P. Godbout. 2015. "Microglial Priming and Enhanced Reactivity to Secondary Insult in Aging, and Traumatic CNS Injury, and Neurodegenerative Disease." *Neuropharmacology* 96:29–41.

O'Connor, M. 2007. *Why Don't Woodpeckers Get Headaches?* Boston: Beacon Press. See p. 177.

Olsen, I. R., R. J. Von Der Heide, K. H. Alm, et al. 2015. "Development of the Uncinate Fasciculus: Implications for Theory and Developmental Disorders." *Developments in Cognitive Neuroscience* 14:50–61.

Ommaya, A. K., and T. A. Gennarelli. 1974. "Cerebral Concussion and Traumatic Unconsciousness: Correlation of Experimental and Clinical Observations on Blunt Head Injuries." *Brain* 97:633–654.

Pearce, A. J., M. Tommerdahl, and D. A. King. 2019. "Neurophysiological Abnormalities in Individuals with Persistent Post-Concussion Symptoms." *Neuroscience* 408:272–281.

Plog, B. A., M. L. Dashnaw, E. Hitomi, et al. 2015. "Biomarkers of Traumatic Injury Are Transported from Brain to Blood via the Glymphatic System." *Journal of Neuroscience* 35(2):518–526.

Povlishock, J. T. 2013. "The Window of Risk in Repeated Head Injury." *Journal of Neurotrauma* 30(1):1.

Prins, M. L., D. Alexander, C. C. Giza, et al. 2013. "Repeated Mild Traumatic Brain Injury: Mechanisms of Cerebral Vulnerability." *Journal of Neurosurgery* 30(1):30–38.

Raam, T., K. M. McAvoy, A. Besnard, et al. 2017. "Hippocampal Oxytocin Receptors Are Necessary for Discrimination of Social Stimuli." *Nature Communications* 8(1):1–14.

Rand, C. W., and C. B. Courville. 1946. "Histologic Changes in the Brain in Cases of Fatal Injury to the Head: VII. Alteration in the Nerve Cells." *Archives of Neurology and Psychiatry* 55(2):79–110. See p. 88.

Romero, K., S. E. Black, and A. Feinstein. 2014. "Differences in Cerebral Perfusion Deficits in Mild Traumatic Brain Injury and Depression Using Single-Photon Emission Computed Tomography." *Frontiers in Neurology* 5:158.

Rowson, S., M. L. Bland, E. T. Campolettano, et al. 2016. "Biomechanical Perspectives on Concussion in Sport." *Sports Medicine and Arthroscopy Review* 24(3):100–107.

Rowson, S., S. M. Duma, J. G. Beckwith, et al. 2012. "Rotational Head Kinematics in Football Impacts: An Injury Risk Function for Concussion." *Annals of Biomedical Engineering* 40(1):1–13.

Scheid, R., D. V. Ott, H. Roth, et al. 2007. "Comparative Magnetic Resonance Imaging at 1.5 and 3 Tesla for the Evaluation of Traumatic Microbleeds." *Journal of Neurotrauma* 24(12):1811–1816.

Seung, S. 2013. *Connectome: How the Brain's Wiring Makes Us Who We Are.* New York: Mariner Press.

Shandra, O., A. R. Winemiller, B. P. Heithoff, et al. 2019. "Repetitive Diffuse Mild Traumatic Brain Injury Causes an Atypical Astrocyte Response and Spontaneous Recurrent Seizures." *Journal of Neuroscience* 39(10):1944–1963.

Sharma, R., A. Rosenberg, E. R. Bennett, et al. 2017. "A Blood-Based Biomarker Panel to Risk-Stratify Mild Traumatic Brain Injury." *PLoS One* 12(3):e0173798.

Shaw, N. A. 2002. "Neurophysiology of Concussion: Theoretical Perspectives." *Progress in Neurobiology* 67:281–344. See p. 283.

Shenton, M. E., H. M. Hamoda, J. S. Schneiderman, et al. 2012. "A Review of Magnetic Resonance Imaging and Diffusion Tensor Imaging Findings in Mild Traumatic Brain Injury." *Brain Imaging and Behavior* 6(2):137–192.

Signoretti, S., G. Lazzarino, B. Tavazzi, et al. 2011. "The Pathophysiology of Concussion." *PM&R* 3(10 suppl. 2):S359–S368.

Signoretti, S., R. Vagnozzi, B. Tavazzi, et al. 2010. "Biochemical and Neurochemical Sequelae Following Mild Traumatic Brain Injury: Summary of Experimental Data and Clinical Implications." *Neurosurgical Focus* 29(5):E1.

Slobounov, S. M., A. Walter, H. C. Breiter, et al. 2017. "The Effect of Repetitive Subconcussive Collisions on Brain Integrity in Collegiate Football Players over a Single Football Season: A Multi-Modality Neuroimaging Study." *Neuroimage: Clinical* 14:708–718.

Strain, J. F., N. Didehbani, C. M. Cullum, et al. 2013. "Depressive Symptoms and White Matter Dysfunction in Retired NFL Players with Concussion History." *Neurology* 81(1):25–32.

Strain, J. F., K. B. Womack, N. Didehbani, et al. 2015. "Imaging Correlates of Memory and Concussion History in Retired National Football Athletes." *JAMA Neurology* 72(7):773–780.

Strich, S. J. 1970. "Lesions in the Cerebral Hemispheres after Blunt Head Injury." *Journal of Clinical Pathology Supplement (Royal College of Pathologists)* 4 (c):166–171.

Tsitsopoulos, P. P., and N. Marklund. 2013. "Amyloid-ß Peptides and Tau Protein as Biomarkers in Cerebrospinal and Interstitial Fluid Following Traumatic Brain Injury: A Review of Experimental and Clinical Studies." *Frontiers in Neurology* 4:79.

Vagnozzi, R., S. Signoretti, L. Cristofori, et al. 2010. "Assessment of Metabolic Brain Damage and Recovery Following Mild Traumatic Brain

Injury: A Multicentre, Proton Magnetic Resonance Spectroscopic Study in Concussed Patients." *Brain* 133(11):3232–3242.

van der Horn, H. J., J. G. Kok, M. E. de Koning, et al. 2017. "Altered Wiring of the Human Structural Connectome in Adults with Mild Traumatic Brain Injury." *Journal of Neurotrauma* 34(5):1035–1044.

Von Der Heide, R. J., L. M. Skipper, E. Klobusicky, et al. 2013. "Dissecting the Uncinate Fasciculus: Disorders, Controversies and a Hypothesis." *Brain* 136(6):1692–1707.

Vos, S. B., M. A. Viergever, and A. Leemans. 2013. "Multi-Fiber Tractography Visualizations for Diffusion MRI Data." *PLoS One* 8(11):e81453.

Wang, L., J. T-M. Cheung, F. Pu, et al. 2011. "Why Do Woodpeckers Resist Head Impact Injury: A Biomechanical Investigation." *PLoS One* 6(10):26490.

Whitaker, K. J., P. E. Vértes, R. Romero-Garcia, et al. 2016. "Adolescence Is Associated with Genomically Patterned Consolidation of the Hubs of the Human Brain Connectome." *Proceedings of the National Academy of Sciences* 113(32):9105–9110.

Windle, W. F., and R. A. Groat. 1945. "Disappearance of Nerve Cells after Concussion." *Anatomic Record* 93:201–209. See p. 202.

Wu, T. C., E. A. Wilde, E. D. Bigler, et al. 2010. "Evaluating the Relationship between Memory Functioning and Cingulum Bundles in Acute Mild Traumatic Brain Injury Using Diffusion Tensor Imaging." *Journal of Neurotrauma* 27(2):303–307.

Yuh, E. L., G. W. J. Hawryluk, and G. T. Manley. 2014. "Imaging Concussion: A Review." *Neurosurgery* 75:S50–63.

Yuh, E. L., P. Mukherjee, H. F. Lingsma, et al. 2013. "Magnetic Resonance Imaging Improves 3-Month Outcome Prediction in Mild Traumatic Brain Injury." *Annals of Neurology* 73(2):224–235.

Zetterberg, H., H. R. Morris, J. Hardy, et al. 2016. "Update on Fluid Biomarkers for Concussion." *Concussion* 1(3):CNC12.

Chapter 2 · The Search for a Diagnosis

Abeare, C. A., I. Messa, B. G. Zuccato, et al. 2018. "Prevalence of Invalid Performance Baseline Testing for Sport-Related Concussion by Age and Validity Indicator." *JAMA Neurology* 75(6):697–703.

Alla, S., S. J. Sullivan, and P. McCrory. 2012. "Defining Asymptomatic Status Following Sports Concussion: Fact or Fallacy?" *British Journal of Sports Medicine* 46(8):562–569.

Allen, B. J., and J. D. Gfeller. 2011. "The Immediate Post-Concussion Assessment and Cognitive Testing Battery and Traditional Neuropsychological Measures: A Construct and Concurrent Validity Study." *Brain Injury* 25(2):179–191.

American Congress of Rehabilitation Medicine. 1993. "Definition of Mild Traumatic Brain Injury." *Journal of Head Trauma Rehabilitation* 8(3):86–87.

Arbogast, K. B., A. E. Curry, M. R. Pfeiffer, et al. 2016. "Point of Health Care Entry for Youth with Concussion within a Large Pediatric Care Network." *JAMA Pediatrics* 170(7):e160294.

Arnett, P., J. Meyer, V. Merritt, et al. 2016. "Neuropsychological Testing in Mild Traumatic Brain Injury." *Sports Medicine and Arthroscopy Review* 24(3):116–122.

Bailes, J. E., A. L. Petraglia, B. I. Omalu, et al. 2013. "Role of Subconcussion in Repetitive Mild Traumatic Brain Injury." *Journal of Neurosurgery* 119(5):1235–1245.

Bailey, C. M., R. J. Echemendia, and P. A. Arnett. 2006. "The Impact of Motivation on Neuropsychological Performance in Sports-Related Mild Traumatic Brain Injury." *Journal of the International Neuropsychological Society* 12(4):475–484.

Balaban, C., M. E. Hoffer, M. Szczupak, et al. 2016. "Oculomotor, Vestibular, and Reaction Time Tests in Mild Traumatic Brain Injury." *PLoS One* 11(9):e0162168.

Belanger, H. G., R. D. Vanderploeg, and T. McAllister. 2016. "Subconcussive Blows to the Head: A Formative Review of Short-Term Clinical Outcomes." *Journal of Head Trauma Rehabilitation* 31(3):159–166.

Börg, J., L. Holm, J. D. Cassidy, et al. 2004. "Diagnostic Procedures in Mild Traumatic Brain Injury: Results of the WHO Collaborating Centre Task Force on Mild Traumatic Brain Injury." *Journal of Rehabilitation Medicine* 36(suppl. 43):61–75.

Broglio, S. P., B. P. Katz, S. Zhao, et al. 2018. "Test-Retest Reliability and Interpretation of Common Concussion Assessment Tools: Findings from the NCAA-DoD Care Consortium." *Sports Medicine* 48: 1255–1268.

Capó-Aponte, J. E., T. A. Beltran, D. V. Walsh, et al. 2018. "Validation of Visual Objective Biomarkers for Acute Concussion." *Military Medicine* 183:9–17.

Carney, N., J. Ghajar, A. Jagoda, et al. 2014. "Concussion Guidelines Step 1: Systematic Review of Prevalent Indicators." *Neurosurgery* 75(3): S3–S15.

Choe, M. C., and C. C. Giza. 2015. "Diagnosis and Management of Acute Concussion." *Seminars in Neurology* 35(1):29–41.

Connery, A. K., R. L. Peterson, D. A. Baker, et al. 2016. "The Role of Neuropsychological Evaluation in the Clinical Management of Concussion." *Physical Medicine and Rehabilitation Clinics of North America* 27(2):475–486.

Denker, P. G. 1954."The Post-Concussion Syndrome: Prognosis and Evaluation of the Organic Factors." *N.Y. State Journal of Medicine* 44:379–384.

Denker, P. G., and G. F. Perry. 1954. "Postconcussion Syndrome in Compensation and Litigation: Analysis of 95 Cases with Electroencephalographic Correlations." *Neurology* 4(12):912–918.

Echemendia, R. J., S. P. Broglio, G. A. Davis, et al. 2017. "What Tests and Measures Should Be Added to the SCAT3 and Related Tests to

Improve Their Reliability, Sensitivity and / or Specificity in Sideline Concussion Diagnosis? A Systematic Review." *British Journal of Sports Medicine* 51(11):895–901.

Edmed, S. L., and K. A. Sullivan. 2014. "Method of Symptom Assessment Influences Cognitive, Affective and Somatic Post-Concussion-Like Symptom Base Rates." *Brain Injury* 28(10):1277–1282.

Eisenberg, M. A., J. Andrea, W. Meehan, et al. 2013. "Time Interval between Concussions and Symptom Duration." *Pediatrics* 132(1):8–17.

Elbin, R. J., J. Knox, N. Kegel, et al. 2016. "Assessing Symptoms in Adolescents Following Sport-Related Concussion: A Comparison of Four Different Approaches." *Applied Neuropsychology: Child* 5(4):294–302.

Ellis, M. J., J. J. Leddy, and B. Willer. 2015. "Physiological, Vestibulo-Ocular and Cervicogenic Post-Concussion Disorders: An Evidence-Based Classification System with Directions for Treatment." *Brain Injury* 29(2):238–248.

Ewing-Cobbs, L., H. S. Levin, J. M. Fletcher, et al. 1990. "The Children's Orientation and Amnesia Test: Relationship to Severity of Acute Head Injury and to Recovery of Memory." *Neurosurgery* 27(5): 683–691.

"FDA Warns Public Not to Use Unapproved or Unclear Medical Devices to Help Assess or Diagnose a Concussion." 2019. Food and Drug Administration, U.S. Health and Human Services, news release, April 10. https://www.fda.gov/NewsEvents/Newsroom/PressAnnouncements /ucm635720.htm.

Gallant, F., J. L. O'Loughlin, J. Brunet, et al. 2017. "Childhood Sports Participation and Adolescent Sport Profile." *Pediatrics* 140(6):e20171449.

Gaudet, C. E., and L. L. Weyandt. 2017. "Immediate Post-Concussion and Cognitive Testing (ImPACT): A Systematic Review of the Prevalence and Assessment of Invalid Performance." *Clinical Neuropsychologist* 31(1):43–58.

Gawande, A. 2009. *The Checklist Manifesto: How to Get Things Right.* New York: Picador Books.

Honce, J. M., E. Nyberg, I. Jones, et al. 2016. "Neuroimaging of Concussion." *Physical Medicine and Rehabilitation Clinics of North America* 27(2):411–428.

Iliad of Homer, The. 1874. Trans. Alexander Pope. London: Frederick Warne. See p. 205.

Iverson, G. L., B. L. Brooks, V. L. Ashton, et al. 2010. "Interview versus Questionnaire Symptom Reporting in People with the Postconcussion Syndrome." *Journal of Head Trauma Rehabilitation* 25(1):23–30.

Iverson, G. L., A. J. Gardner, D. P. Terry, et al. 2017. "Predictors of Clinical Recovery from Concussion: A Systematic Review." *British Journal of Sports Medicine* 51(12):941–948.

Iverson, G. L., N. D. Silverberg, R. Mannix, et al. 2015. "Factors Associated with Concussion-like Symptom Reporting in High School Athletes." *JAMA Pediatrics* 169(12):1132–1140.

Jagoda, A. S., J. J. Bazarian, J. J. Bruns, et al. 2008. "Clinical Policy: Neuroimaging and Decision-making in Adult Mild Traumatic Brain Injury in the Acute Setting." *Annals of Emergency Medicine* 52(6):714–748.

Kay, D. W. K., T. A. Kerr, and L. P. Lassman. 1971. "Brain Trauma and the Post-Concussional Syndrome." *Lancet* 298(7733):1052–1055. See p. 1055.

Kelly, R. 1975. "The Post-Traumatic Syndrome: An Iatrogenic Disease." *Forensic Science* 6:17–24. See p. 23–24.

Kelly, R. 1981. "Post-Traumatic Syndrome." *Journal of the Royal Society of Medicine* 74:242–244.

Kelly, R., and B. N. Smith. 1981."Post-Traumatic Syndrome: Another Myth Discredited." *Journal of the Royal Society of Medicine* 74:275–277. See p. 275.

Kenzie, E. S., E. L. Parks, E. D. Bigler, et al. 2017. "Concussion as a Multi-Scale Complex System: An Interdisciplinary Synthesis of Current Knowledge." *Frontiers in Neurology* 8:513.

Kumar, S., A. Jawahar, and P. Shah. 2015. "Montreal Cognitive Assessment, a Screening Tool for Mild Traumatic Brain Injury." *Neurology* 84(14 suppl.):P7.185.

Leddy, J. J., J. G. Baker, A. Merchant, et al. 2015. "Brain or Strain? Symptoms Alone Do Not Distinguish Physiologic Concussion from Cervical / Vestibular Injury." *Clinical Journal of Sports Medicine* 25(3):237–242.

Levin, H. S., V. M. O'Donnell, and R. G. Grossman. 1979. "The Galveston Orientation and Amnesia Test: A Practical Scale to Assess Cognition after Head Injury." *Journal of Nervous and Mental Diseases* 167(11):675–684.

Lidvall, H. F., B. Linderoth, and B. Norton. 1974. "Causes of the Post-Concussional Syndrome." *Acta Neurologica Scandinavia* 50(suppl. 56):64–71.

Marshall, C. M., H. Vernon, J. J. Leddy, et al. 2015. "The Role of the Cervical Spine in Post-Concussion Syndrome." *Physician and Sports Medicine* 43(3):274–284.

Matuszak, J. M., J. McVige, J. McPherson, et al. 2016. "A Practical Concussion Physical Examination Toolbox: Evidence-Based Physical Examination for Concussion." *Sports Health* 8(3):260–269.

McCrea M., T. Hammeke, G. Olsen, et al. 2004. "Unreported Concussion in High School Football Players: Implications for Prevention." *Clinical Journal of Sports Medicine* 14:13–17.

Miller, H. 1961. "Accident Neurosis." *British Medical Journal* 1(5230):919–925. See pp. 919 and 922.

Mucha, A., M. W. Collins, R. J. Elbin, et al. 2014. "A Brief Vestibular / Ocular Motor Screening (VOMS) Assessment to Evaluate Concussions: Preliminary Findings." *American Journal of Sports Medicine* 42(10):2479–2486.

Narad, M., M. Kennelly, N. Zhang, et al. 2018. "Secondary Attention-Deficit/Hyperactivity Disorder in Children and Adolescents 5 to 10 Years after Traumatic Brain Injury." *JAMA Pediatrics* 172(5): 437–443.

Nichols, A. H. 1886. "Alleged Organic Disease of the Brain Following Moderate Concussion—Case of Louisa V. Russell vs. Boston & Lowell R.R. Company." *Boston Medicine and Surgery Journal* 114:509–511. See pp. 510 and 511.

Ott, S. D., C. M. Bailey, and D. K. Broshek. 2018. "An Interdisciplinary Approach to Sports Concussion Evaluation and Management: The Role of a Neuropsychologist." *Archives of Clinical Neuropsychology* 33(3):319–329.

Pape, T. L.-B., W. M. High, J. St. Andre, et al. 2013. "Diagnostic Accuracy Studies in Mild Traumatic Brain Injury: A Systematic Review and Descriptive Analysis of Published Evidence." *PM&R* 5(10):856–881.

Patricios, J., G. W. Fuller, R. Ellenbogen, et al. 2017. "What Are the Critical Elements of Sideline Screening That Can Be Used to Establish the Diagnosis of Concussion? A Systematic Review." *British Journal of Sports Medicine* 51(11):888–894.

Pillai, C., and J. W. Gittinger. 2017. "Vision Testing in the Evaluation of Concussion." *Seminars in Ophthalmology* 32(1):144–152.

Podell, K., C. Presley, and H. Derman. 2017. "Sideline Sports Concussion Assessment." *Neurologic Clinics* 35(3):435–450.

Ponsford, J., P. Cameron, M. Fitzgerald, et al. 2012. "Predictors of Postconcussive Symptoms 3 Months after Mild Traumatic Brain Injury." *Neuropsychology* 26(3):304–313.

Prince, C., and M. E. Bruhns. 2017. "Evaluation and Treatment of Mild Traumatic Brain Injury: The Role of Neuropsychology." *Brain Sciences* 7(8):105.

Prins, A., M. J. Bovin, R. Kimerling, et al. 2015. "Primary Care PTSD Screen for DSM-5 (PC-PTSD-5) [Measurement Instrument]."

https://www.ptsd.va.gov/professional/assessment/documents/pc-ptsd5-screen.pdf.

Putukian, M. 2011. "Neuropsychological Testing as It Relates to Recovery from Sports-Related Concussion." *PM&R* 3(10 suppl. 2):S425–S432.

Reddy, C. C. 2011. "Postconcussion Syndrome: A Physiatrist's Approach." *PM&R* 3(10 suppl. 2):S396–S405.

Register-Mihalik, J. K., and M. C. Kay. 2017. "The Current State of Sports Concussion." *Neurologic Clinics* 35(3):387–402.

Reneker, J. C., V. K. Cheruvu, J. Yang, et al. 2017. "Physical Examination of Dizziness in Athletes after a Concussion: A Descriptive Study." *Musculoskeletal Science and Practice* 34:8–13.

Ross, R. 2018. "Between Shell Shock and PTSD? 'Accident Neuroses' and Its Sequelae in Post-War Britain." *Social History of Medicine* 32(3):565–585. See p. 575.

Ruff, R. M. 2011. "Mild Traumatic Brain Injury and Neural Recovery: Rethinking the Debate." *NeuroRehabilitation* 28(3):167–180.

Ruff, R. M., G. L. Iverson, J. T. Barth, et al. 2009. "Recommendations for Diagnosing a Mild Traumatic Brain Injury: A National Academy of Neuropsychology Education Paper." *Archives of Clinical Neuropsychology* 24(1):3–10.

Russell, W. R. 1961. "Post-Traumatic Amnesia in Closed Head Injury." *Archives of Neurology* 5:16–29. See p. 27.

———. 1964. "Some Reactions of the Nervous System to Trauma." *British Medical Journal* 2(5406):403–407.

Rutherford, W. H., J. D. Merrett, and J. R. McDonald. 1977. "Sequelae of Concussion Caused by Minor Head Injuries." *Lancet* 1(8001):1–4. See p. 4.

———. 1978. "Symptoms at One Year Following Concussion from Minor Head Injuries." *Injury* 10:225–230. See p. 230.

Samadani, U., R. R. M. Eng, M. Reyes, et al. 2015. "Eye Tracking Detects Disconjugate Eye Movements Associated with Structural Traumatic Brain Injury and Concussion." *Journal of Neurotrauma* 32(8):548–556.

Sherer, M., M. A. Struchen, S. A. Yablon, et al. 2008. "Comparison of Indices of Traumatic Brain Injury Severity: Glasgow Coma Scale, Length of Coma and Post-traumatic Amnesia." *Journal of Neurology, Neurosurgery and Psychiatry* 79(6):678–685.

Silver, J. M. 2012. "Effort, Exaggeration and Malingering after Concussion." *Journal of Neurology, Neurosurgery and Psychiatry* 83(8):836–841, p. 839.

Sussman, E. S., A. L. Ho, A. V. Pendharkar, et al. 2016. "Clinical Evaluation of Concussion: The Evolving Role of Oculomotor Assessments." *Neurosurgical Focus* 40(4):E7.

Taylor, A. R. 1967. "Post-Concussional Sequelae." *British Medical Journal* 3:67–71. See p. 67.

Teasdale, G., and B. Jennett. 1974. "Assessment of Impaired Consciousness and Coma: A Practical Scale." *Lancet* 2:81–82.

Teel, E. F., M. R. Gay, P. A. Arnett, et al. 2016. "Differential Sensitivity between a Virtual Reality Balance Module and Clinically Used Concussion Balance Modalities." *Clinical Journal of Sport Medicine* 26(2):162–166.

Torres, D. M., K. M. Galetta, H. W. Phillips, et al. 2013. "Sports-Related Concussion: Anonymous Survey of a Collegiate Cohort." *Neurology: Clinical Practice* 3(4):279–287.

Ventura, R. E., L. J. Balcer, and S. L. Galetta. 2014. "The Neuro-Ophthalmology of Head Trauma." *Lancet Neurology* 13(10):1006–1016.

———. 2015. "The Concussion Toolbox: The Role of Vision in the Assessment of Concussion." *Seminars in Neurology* 35(5):599–606.

Ventura, R. E., L. J. Balcer, S. L. Galetta, et al. 2016. "Ocular Motor Assessment in Concussion: Current Status and Future Directions." *Journal of the Neurological Sciences* 361:79–86.

von Brevern, M., and T. Lempert. 2001. "Benign Paroxysmal Positional Vertigo." *Archives of Neurology* 58:1491–1493.

Wallace, B., and J. Lifshitz. 2016. "Traumatic Brain Injury and Vestibulo-Ocular Function: Current Challenges and Future Prospects." *Eye and Brain* 8:153–164.

World Health Organization: The ICD-10 Classification of Mental and Behavioural Disorders: Clinical Descriptions and Diagnostic Guidelines. Geneva, World Health Organization, 1992.

Chapter 3 ▪ Concussion Care

Austen, J. 1933. *The Novels of Jane Austen,* vol. 5: *Northanger Abbey and Persuasion,* 3rd ed. Ed. R. W. Chapman. Oxford: Oxford University Press. See pp. 109 and 218.

Baker, J. G., M. S. Freitas, J. J. Leddy, et al. 2012. "Return to Full Functioning after Graded Exercise Assessment and Progressive Exercise Treatment of Postconcussion Syndrome." *Rehabilitation Research and Practice:* Epub 705309.

Baumann, C. R. 2016. "Sleep and Traumatic Brain Injury." *Sleep Medicine Clinics* 11(1):19–23.

Blume, H. K. 2015. "Headaches after Concussion in Pediatrics: A Review." *Current Pain and Headache Reports* 19(9):1–11.

Brown, A. W., T. K. Watanabe, J. M. Hoffman, et al. 2015. "Headache after Traumatic Brain Injury: A National Survey of Clinical Practices and Treatment Approaches." *PM&R* 7(1):3–8.

Brown, N. J., R. C. Mannix, M. J. O'Brien, et al. 2014. "Effect of Cognitive Activity Level on Duration of Post-Concussion Symptoms." *Pediatrics* 133(2):e299–304.

Centers for Disease Control and Prevention. 2012. "Short Sleep Duration among Workers—United States, 2010." *Morbidity and Mortality Weekly Report* 61(16):281–285.

Chrisman, S. P. D., and L. P. Richardson. 2014. "Prevalence of Diagnosed Depression in Adolescents with History of Concussion." *Journal of Adolescent Health* 54(5):582–586.

Chrisman, S. P. D., and F. P. Rivara. 2016. "Physical Activity or Rest after Concussion in Youth: Questions about Timing and Potential Benefit." *JAMA* 316(23):2491–2492.

DiFazio, M., N. D. Silverberg, M. W. Kirkwood, et al. 2015. "Prolonged Activity Restriction after Concussion: Are We Worsening Outcomes?" *Clinical Pediatrics* 55(5):443–451.

Engel, G. L. 1980. "The Biopsychosocial Model." *American Journal of Psychiatry* 137(5):535–544.

Freeman, M. D., S. Rosa, D. Harshfield, et al. 2010. "A Case-Control Study of Cerebellar Tonsillar Ectopia (Chiari) and Head / Neck Trauma (Whiplash)." *Brain Injury* 24(7–8):988–994.

Giza, C. C., M. C. Choe, and K. M. Barlow. 2018. "Determining If Rest Is Best after Concussion." *JAMA Neurology* 75(4):399–400.

Grool, A. M., M. Aglipay, F. Momoli, et al. 2016. "Association between Early Participation in Physical Activity Following Acute Concussion and Persistent Postconcussive Symptoms in Children and Adolescents." *JAMA* 316(23): 2504–2514.

Halstead, M. E., K. D. Walter, and K. Moffett. 2018. "Sport Related Concussion in Children and Adolescents." *Pediatrics* 142(6):e2018 3074.

Hershey, A. D. 2017. "CGRP—The Next Frontier for Migraine." *New England Journal of Medicine* 377(22):2190–2191.

Hesse, G. 2016. "Evidence and Evidence Gaps in Tinnitus Therapy." *Current Topics in Otorhinolaryngology—Head and Neck Surgery* 15:1–42.

Iverson, G. L., and G. A. Gioia. 2016. "Returning to School Following Sport-Related Concussion." *Physical Medicine and Rehabilitation Clinics of North America* 27(2):429–436.

Jonas, W. B., D. M. Bellanti, C. F. Paat, et al. 2016. "A Randomized Exploratory Study to Evaluate Two Acupuncture Methods for the Treatment of Headaches Associated with Traumatic Brain Injury." *Medical Acupuncture* 28(3):113–130.

Kerr, Z., S. L. Zuckerman, E. B. Wasserman, et al. 2016. "Concussion Symptoms and Return to Play Time in Youth, High School, and College American Football Athletes." *JAMA Pediatrics* 170(7): 647–653.

Leddy, J., A. Hinds, D. Sirica, et al. 2016. "The Role of Controlled Exercise in Concussion Management." *PM&R* 8(3):S91–S100.

Lucas, S., J. M. Hoffman, K. R. Bell, et al. 2014. "A Prospective Study of Prevalence and Characterization of Headache Following Mild Traumatic Brain Injury." *Cephalalgia* 34(2):93–102.

McCrory, P., W. H. Meeuwisse, M. Aubry, et al. 2013. "Consensus Statement on Concussion in Sport: The 4th International Conference on Concussion in Sport Held in Zurich, November 2012." *British Journal of Sports Medicine* 47(5):250–258.

McCrory, P., W. Meeuwisse, J. Dvořák, et al. 2017. "Consensus Statement on Concussion in Sport: The 5th International Conference on Concussion in Sport Held in Berlin, October 2016." *British Journal of Sports Medicine* 51(11):838–847. See p. 842.

Miele, V. J., J. E. Bailes, and N. A. Martin. 2006. "Participation in Contact or Collision Sports in Athletes with Epilepsy, Genetic Risk Factors, Structural Brain Lesions, or History of Craniotomy." *Neurosurgery Focus* 21(4):E9.

Morawska, M. M., F. Buchele, C. G. Moreira, et al. 2016. "Sleep Modulation Alleviates Axonal Damage and Cognitive Decline after Rodent Traumatic Brain Injury." *Journal of Neuroscience* 36(12):3422–3429.

Murray, D. A., D. Meldrum, and O. Lennon. 2017. "Can Vestibular Rehabilitation Exercises Help Patients with Concussion? A Systematic Review of Efficacy, Prescription and Progression Patterns." *British Journal of Sports Medicine* 51(5):442–451.

O'Brien, M. J., D. R. Howell, M. J. Pepin, et al. 2017. "Sport-Related Concussions: Symptom Recurrence after Return to Exercise." *Orthopaedic Journal of Sports Medicine* 5(10):1–6.

Ouellet, M.-C., S. Beaulieu-Bonneau, and C. M. Morin. 2015. "Sleep-Wake Disturbances after Traumatic Brain Injury." *Lancet Neurology* 14(7):746–757.

Phillips, M. M., and C. C. Reddy. 2016. "Managing Patients with Prolonged Recovery Following Concussion." *Physical Medicine and Rehabilitation Clinics of North America* 27:455–474.

Ponsford, J., C. Willmont, A. Rothwell, et al. 2002. "Impact of Early Intervention on Outcome Following Mild Head Injury in Adults." *Journal of Neurology, Neurosurgery, and Psychiatry* 73:330–332.

Ponsford, J. L., and K. L. Sinclair. 2014. "Sleep and Fatigue Following Traumatic Brain Injury." *Psychiatric Clinics of North America* 37(1): 77–89.

Radhakrishnan, R., A. Garakani, L. S. Gross, et al. 2016. "Neuropsychiatric Aspects of Concussion." *Lancet Psychiatry* 3(12):1166–1175.

Sandsmark, D. K., J. E. Elliott, and M. M. Lim. 2017. "Sleep-Wake Disturbances after Traumatic Brain Injury: Synthesis of Human and Animal Studies." *Sleep: Journal of Sleep and Sleep Disorders Research* 40(5):1–18.

Sawyer, Q., B. Vesci, and T. C. V. McLeod. 2016. "Physical Activity and Intermittent Postconcussion Symptoms after a Period of Symptom-Limited Physical and Cognitive Rest." *Journal of Athletic Training* 51(9):739–742.

Schneider, K. J., J. J. Leddy, K. M. Guskiewicz, et al. 2017. "Rest and Treatment / Rehabilitation Following Sport-Related Concussion: A Systematic Review." *British Journal of Sports Medicine* 51:930–934.

Semple, B. D., S. Lee, R. Sadjadi, et al. 2015. "Repetitive Concussions in Adolescent Athletes: Translating Clinical and Experimental Research into Perspectives on Rehabilitation Strategies." *Frontiers in Neurology* 6:69.

Silver, J. M. 2014. "Neuropsychiatry of Persistent Symptoms after Concussion." *Psychiatric Clinics of North America* 37(1):91–102.

Silverberg, N. D., G. L. Iverson, M. McCrea, et al. 2016. "Activity-Related Symptom Exacerbations after Pediatric Concussion." *JAMA Pediatrics* 170(10):946–953.

Singh, K., A. M. Morse, N. Tkachenko, et al. 2016. "Sleep Disorders Associated with Traumatic Brain Injury: A Review." *Pediatric Neurology* 60:30–36.

Stacey, A., S. Lucas, S. Dikmen, et al. 2017. "Natural History of Headache Five Years after Traumatic Brain Injury." *Journal of Neurotrauma* 34(8):1558–1564.

Stein, M. B., and T. W. McAllister. 2009. "Exploring the Convergence of Posttraumatic Stress Disorder and Mild Traumatic Brain Injury." *American Journal of Psychiatry* 166(7):768–776.

Sullivan-Singh, S. J., K. Sawyer, D. M. Ehde, et al. 2014. "Comorbidity of Pain and Depression among Persons with Traumatic Brain Injury." *Archives of Physical Medicine and Rehabilitation* 95(6):1100–1105.

Theeler, B., S. Lucas, R. G. Riechers, et al. 2013. "Post-Traumatic Headaches in Civilians and Military Personnel: A Comparative, Clinical Review." *Headache* 53(6):881–900.

Thiagarajan, P., K. J. Ciuffreda, J. E. Capó-Aponte, et al. 2014. "Oculomotor Neurorehabilitation for Reading in Mild Traumatic Brain Injury (MTBI): An Integrative Approach." *NeuroRehabilitation* 34(1):129–146.

Thomas, D. G., J. N. Apps, R. G. Hoffmann, et al. 2015. "Benefits of Strict Rest after Acute Concussion: A Randomized Controlled Trial." *Pediatrics* 135(2):213–223.

Varner, C. E., S. McLeod, N. Nahiddi, et al. 2017. "Cognitive Rest and Graduated Return to Usual Activities versus Usual Care for Mild Traumatic Brain Injury: A Randomized Controlled Trial of Emergency Department Discharge Instructions." *Academic Emergency Medicine* 24(1):75–82.

Wan, M. J., H. Nomura, and C. H. Tator. 2008. "Conversion to Symptomatic Chiari I Malformation after Minor Head or Neck Trauma." *Neurosurgery* 63(4):748–753.

Chapter 4 · Long-Term Risks

Asken, B. M., M. J. Sullan, S. T. DeKosky, et al. 2017. "Research Gaps and Controversies in Chronic Traumatic Encephalopathy: A Review." *JAMA Neurology* 74(10):1255–1262.

Barrio, J. R., G. W. Small, K-P. Wong, et al. 2015. "In Vivo Characterization of Chronic Traumatic Encephalopathy Using [F-18]FDDNP PET Brain Imaging." *Proceedings of the National Academy of Sciences* 112(16):E2039–2047.

Belson, K. 2017. "Aaron Hernandez Found to Have Severe C.T.E." *New York Times,* September 21.

———. 2018. "He Helped Ex-Players Get Benefits. His Family Is Still Waiting." *New York Times,* January 13.

Bieniek, K. F., M. M. Blessing, M. G. Heckman, et al. 2019. "Association between Contact Sports Participation and Chronic Traumatic Encephalopathy: A Retrospective Cohort Study." *Brain Pathology:* https://doi.org/10.1111/bpa.12757.

Bowman, K. M., and A. Blau. 1940. "Psychotic States Following Head and Brain Injury in Adults and Children." In *Injuries of the Skull, Brain and Spinal Cord: Neuro-psychiatric, Surgical and Medio-Legal Aspects,* ed. S. Brock, 309–360. Baltimore, MD: Williams and Wilkins.

Bryan, M. A., A. Rowhani-Rahbar, R. D. Comstock, et al. 2016. "Sports- and Recreation-Related Concussions in US Youth." *Pediatrics* 138(1):e20154635.

Carroll, L. J., J. D. Cassidy, C. Cancelliere, et al. 2014. "Systematic Review of the Prognosis after Mild Traumatic Brain Injury in Adults: Cognitive, Psychiatric, and Mortality Outcomes: Results of the International Collaboration on Mild Traumatic Brain Injury Prognosis." *Archives of Physical Medicine and Rehabilitation* 95(3 suppl.2):S152–S173.

Casper, S. 2018. "Concussion: A History of Science and Medicine, 1870–2005." *Headache* 58:795–810.

Centers for Disease Control and Prevention, National Institute for Occupational Safety and Health (NIOSH). 1994. National Football League Players Mortality Study. Cincinnati, OH: NIOSH. *Health Hazard Evaluation,* 88-085.

Chandler, A. 2015. "Frank Gifford and the NFL's Concussion Crisis." *Atlantic.* November 25.

Chen, Y.-H., J. J. Keller, J.-H. Kang, et al. 2012. "Association between Traumatic Brain Injury and the Subsequent Risk of Brain Cancer." *Journal of Neurotrauma* 29(7):1328–1333.

Cherry, J. D., Y. Tripodis, V. E. Alvarez, et al. 2016. "Microglial Neuroinflammation Contributes to Tau Accumulation in Chronic Traumatic Encephalopathy." *Acta Neuropathologica Communications* 4(1):112.

Corsellis, J. A. N. 1989. "Boxing and the Brain." *British Medical Journal* 298:105–109.

Crane, P. K., L. E. Gibbons, K. Dams-O'Connor, et al. 2016. "Association of Traumatic Brain Injury with Late-Life Neurodegenerative Conditions and Neuropathologic Findings." *JAMA Neurology* 73(9):1062–1069.

Critchley, M. 1957. "Medical Aspects of Boxing, Particularly from a Neurological Standpoint." *British Medical Journal* 1(5015):357–362.

Davidson, J., M. D. Cusimano, and W. G. Bendena. 2015. "Post-Traumatic Brain Injury: Genetic Susceptibility to Outcome." *Neuroscientist* 21(4):424–441.

Deutsch, M. B., M. F. Mendez, and E. Teng. 2015. "Interactions between Traumatic Brain Injury and Frontotemporal Degeneration." *Dementia and Geriatric Cognitive Disorders* 39(0):143–153.

Faden, A. I., and D. J. Loane. 2015. "Chronic Neurodegeneration after Traumatic Brain Injury: Alzheimer Disease, Chronic Traumatic Encephalopathy, or Persistent Neuroinflammation?" *Neurotherapeutics* 12(1):143–150.

Fainaru, S., and M. Fainaru-Wada. 2019. "For the NFL and All of Football, a New Threat: An Evaporating Insurance Market." ESPN.com, January 17. http://www.espn.com/espn/print?id=25776964.

Fiore, C. 2016. "'The Great DeKosky' Talks CTE and Concussion." *MedPage Today,* January 14.

"Football Player's Safe Exit, A." 2016. Editorial, *New York Times,* March 22.

Gardner, A., G. L. Iverson, and P. McCrory. 2014. "Chronic Traumatic Encephalopathy in Sport: A Systematic Review." *British Journal of Sports Medicine* 48:84–90.

Gardner, R. C., J. F. Burke, J. Nettiksimmons, et al. 2014. "Dementia Risk after Traumatic Brain Injury vs Nonbrain Trauma: The Role of Age and Severity." *JAMA Neurology* 71(12):1490–1497.

Gardner, R. C., J. F. Burke, J. Nettiksimmons, et al. 2015. "Traumatic Brain Injury in Later Life Increases Risk for Parkinson's Disease." *Annals of Neurology* 77(6):987–995.

Geddes, J. F., G. H. Vowles, J. A. Nicoll, et al. 1999. "Neuronal Cytoskeletal Changes Are an Early Consequence of Repetitive Head Injury." *Acta Neuropathologica* 98(2):171–178.

Gedye, A., B. L. Beattie, H. Tuokko, et al. 1989. "Severe Head Injury Hastens Early Onset of Alzheimer's Disease." *Journal of the American Geriatrics Society* 37(10):970–973.

Godbolt, A. K., C. Cancelliere, C A. Hincapié, et al. 2014. "Systematic Review of the Risk of Dementia and Chronic Cognitive Impairment after Mild Traumatic Brain Injury: Results of the International Collaboration on Mild Traumatic Brain Injury Prognosis." *Archives of Physical Medicine and Rehabilitation* 95(3 suppl. 2):S245–S256.

Grashow, R., M. G. Weisskopf, K. K. Miller, et al. 2019. "Erectile Dysfunction in Professional US-Style Football Players." *JAMA Neurology.* August 26. doi:10.1001/jamaneurol.2019.2664.

Guo, Z., L. A. Cupples, A. Kurz, et al. 2000. "Head Injury and the Risk of AD in the MIRAGE Study." *Neurology* 54(6):1316–1323.

Guskiewicz, K. M., S. W. Marshall, J. Bailes, et al. 2005. "Association between Recurrent Concussion and Late-Life Cognitive Impairment in Retired Professional Football Players." *Neurosurgery* 57(4):719–726.

Guttman, A. 2006. "Civilized Mayhem: Origins and Early Development of American Football." *Sport in Society* 9(4):533–541. See p. 536.

Harrison, E. A. 2014. "The First Concussion Crisis: Head Injury and Evidence in Early American Football." *American Journal of Public Health* 104(5):822–833. See p. 825.

Hayes, J. P., M. W. Logue, N. Sadeh, et al. 2017. "Mild Traumatic Brain Injury Is Associated with Reduced Cortical Thickness in Those at Risk for Alzheimer's Disease." *Brain* 140:813–825.

Hernandez, J. 2018. *The Truth About Aaron: My Journey to Understand My Brother.* New York: Barnes and Noble.

Himanen, L., R. Portin, H. Isoniemi, et al. 2006. "Longitudinal Cognitive Changes in Traumatic Brain Injury." *Neurology* 66:187–192.

Iverson, G. L., C. D. Keene, G. Perry, et al. 2018. "The Need to Separate Chronic Traumatic Encephalopathy Neuropathology from Clinical Features." *Journal of Alzheimer's Disease* 61(1):17–28.

Jafari, S., M. Etminan, F. Aminzadeh, et al. 2013. "Head Injury and Risk of Parkinson Disease: A Systematic Review and Meta-Analysis." *Movement Disorders* 28(9):1222–1229.

Jordan, B. D. 2000. "Chronic Traumatic Brain Injury Associated with Boxing." *Seminars in Neurology* 20(2):179–186.

Jordan, B. D., N. R. Relkin, L. D. Ravdin, et al. 1997. "Apolipoprotein E Epsilon4 Associated with Chronic Traumatic Brain Injury in Boxing." *JAMA* 278(2):136–140.

Kirkman, M., and A. F. Albert. 2012. "Traumatic Brain Injury and Subsequent Risk of Developing Brain Tumors." *Journal of Neurotrauma* 29(13):2365–2366.

Koerte, I. K., J. Hufschmidt, M. Muehlmann, et al. 2016. "Cavum Septi Pellucidi in Symptomatic Former Professional Football Players." *Journal of Neurotrauma* 33(4):346–353.

Koerte, I. K., A. P. Lin, A. Willems, et al. 2015. "A Review of Neuroimaging Findings in Repetitive Brain Trauma." *Brain Pathology* 25(3):318–349.

Kondo, A., K. Shahpasand, R. Mannix, et al. 2015. "Cis p-Tau: Early Driver of Brain Injury and Tauopathy Blocked by Antibody." *Nature* 523(7561):431–436.

Laskas, J. M. 2015. *Concussion*. New York: Random House. See p. 134.

Lawrence, D. W., P. Comper, M. G. Hutchison, et al. 2015. "The Role of Apolipoprotein E Epsilon (ε)-4 Allele on Outcome Following Traumatic Brain Injury: A Systematic Review." *Brain Injury* 29(9):1018–1031.

Lehman, E. J. 2013. "Epidemiology of Neurodegeneration in American-Style Professional Football Players" *Alzheimer's Research and Therapy* 5(4):34.

Ling, H., H. R. Morris, J. W. Neal, et al. 2017. "Mixed Pathologies Including Chronic Traumatic Encephalopathy Account for Dementia in Retired Association Football (Soccer) Players." *Acta Neuropathologica* 133(3):337–352.

Liu, S-W., L-C. Huang, W-F. Chung, et al. 2017. "The Increased Risk of Stroke in Patients of Concussion: A National Cohort Study." *International Journal of Environmental Research and Public Health* 14(230):1–12.

Lucke-Wold, B. P., R. C. Turner, A. F. Logsdon, et al. 2016. "Endoplasmic Reticulum Stress Implicated in Chronic Traumatic Encephalopathy." *Journal of Neurosurgery* 124:687–702.

Lunny, C. A., S. N. Fraser, and J. A. Knopp-Sihota. 2014. "Physical Trauma and Risk of Multiple Sclerosis: A Systematic Review and Meta-Analysis of Observational Studies." *Journal of the Neurological Sciences* 336:13–23.

"Madness of Sport, The." 1915 / 2014. Editorial, *JAMA* 65(25)2168–2169. Reprinted *JAMA* 314(23):2572.

Manley, G. T., A. J. Gardner, K. J. Schneider, et al. 2017. "A Systematic Review of Potential Long-Term Effects of Sport-Related Concussion." *British Journal of Sports Medicine* 51(12):969–977. See p. 975.

Maroon, J. C., R. Winkelman, and J. Bost. 2015. "Chronic Traumatic Encephalopathy in Contact Sports: A Systematic Review of All Reported Pathological Cases." *PLoS One* 10(2): 1–16.

Marras, C., C. A. Hincapié, V. L. Kristman, et al. 2014. "Systematic Review of the Risk of Parkinson's Disease after Mild Traumatic Brain Injury: Results of the International Collaboration on Mild Traumatic Brain Injury Prognosis." *Archives of Physical Medicine and Rehabilitation* 95(3 suppl.):238–244. See p. 238.

Martland, H. S. 1928. "Punch Drunk." *Journal of the American Medical Association* 91(15):1103–1107. See p. 1103.

McKee, A. C., N. J. Cairns, D. W. Dickson, et al. 2016. "The First NINDS / NIBIB Consensus Meeting to Define Neuropathological Criteria for the Diagnosis of Chronic Traumatic Encephalopathy." *Acta Neuropathologica* 131(1):75–86.

McKee, A. C., T. D. Stein, and P. T. Kiernan. 2015. "The Neuropathology of Chronic Traumatic Encephalopathy." *Brain Pathology* 25(3):350–364.

Merritt, V. C., and P. A. Arnett. 2016. "Apolipoprotein E. Apolipoprotein E (APOE) ε4 Allele is Associated with Increased Symptom Reporting Following Sports Concussion." *Journal of the International Neuropsychology Society* 22:89–94.

Mez, J., D. H. Daneshvar, P. T. Kiernan, et al. 2017. "Clinicopathological Evaluation of Chronic Traumatic Encephalopathy in Players of American Football." *JAMA* 318(4):360–370.

Miller, H. 1966. "Mental Sequelae of Head Injury." *Proceedings of the Royal Society of Medicine* 59:257–261.

Millspaugh, J. 1937. "Dementia Pugilistica." *US Naval Medical Bulletin* 35:297–303.

Montenigro, P. H., D. T. Corp, T. D. Stein, et al. 2015. "Chronic Traumatic Encephalopathy: Historical Origins and Current Perspective." *Annual Review of Clinical Psychology* 11:309–330.

Montgomery, S., A. Hiyoshi, and S. Burkill. 2017. "Concussion in Adolescence and Risk of MS." *Annals of Neurology* 82(4):554–561.

Namjoshi, D. R., W. H. Cheng, M. Carr, et al. 2016. "Chronic Exposure to Androgenic-Anabolic Steroids Exacerbates Axonal Injury and Microgliosis in the CHIMERA Mouse Model of Repetitive Concussion." *PLoS One* 11(1):e0146540.

Nemetz, P. N., C. Leibson, J. M. Naessens, et al. 1999. "Traumatic Brain Injury and Time to Onset of Alzheimer's Disease: A Population-based Study." *American Journal of Epidemiology* 149(1):32–40.

Nichols, E. H., and H. B. Smith. 1906. "The Physical Aspect of American Football." *Boston Medicine and Surgical Journal* 154(1):1–8.

Nordström, P., K. Michaelsson, Y. Gustafson, et al. 2014. "Traumatic Brain Injury and Young Onset Dementia: A Nationwide Cohort Study." *Annals of Neurology* 75(3):374–381.

Nordström, A., and P. Nordström. 2018. "Traumatic Brain Injury and the Risk of Dementia Diagnosis: A Nationwide Cohort Study." *PLoS Med* 15(1):e1002496.

Omalu, B., G. W. Small, J. Bailes, et al. 2018. "Postmortem Autopsy-Confirmation of Antemortem [F-18] FDDNP-PET Scans in a Football Player with Chronic Traumatic Encephalopathy." *Clinical Neurosurgery* 82(2):237–246.

Omalu, B. I., S. T. DeKosky, R. L. Hamilton, et al. 2006. "Chronic Traumatic Encephalopathy in a National Football League Player: Part II." *Neurosurgery* 59(5):1086–1092.

Omalu, B. I., S. T. DeKosky, R. L. Minster, et al. 2005. "Chronic Traumatic Encephalopathy in a National Football League Player." *Neurosurgery* 57(1):128–133.

Orlovska, S., M. S. Pedersen, M. E. Benros, et al. 2014. "Head Injury as Risk Factor for Psychiatric Disorders: A Nationwide Register-Based

Follow-Up Study of 113,906 Persons with Head Injury." *American Journal of Psychiatry* 171(4):463–469.

Osnato, M. 1930. "The Role of Trauma in Various Neuropsychiatric Conditions." *American Journal of Psychiatry* 86(4):646–660.

Osnato, M., and V. Giliberti. 1927. "Post-Concussion Neurosis—Traumatic Encephalitis: A Conception of Postconcussion Phenomena." *Archives of Neurology and Psychiatry* 18:181–214.

Parker, H. L. 1934. "Traumatic Encephalopathy ('Punch Drunk') of Professional Pugilists." *Journal of Neurology and Neuropathology* 15:30–34.

Perry, D. C., V. E. Sturm, M. J. Peterson, et al. 2016. "Association of Traumatic Brain Injury with Neurological and Psychiatric Disease: A Meta-Analysis." *Journal of Neurosurgery* 124(2):511–526.

Preston-Martin, S., J. M. Pogoda, B. Schlehofer, et al. 1998. "An International Case-Control Study of Adult Glioma and Meningioma: The Role of Head Trauma." *International Journal of Epidemiology* 27(4):579–586.

Rabinovici, G. D. 2017. "Advances and Gaps in Understanding Chronic Traumatic Encephalopathy: From Pugilists to American Football Players." *Journal of the American Medical Society* 318(4):338–340. See p. 339.

Reams, N., J. T. Eckner, A. A. Almeida, et al. 2016. "A Clinical Approach to the Diagnosis of Traumatic Encephalopathy Syndrome." *JAMA Neurology* 73(6):743–749.

Roberts, A. H. 1969. *Brain Damage in Boxers: A Study of the Prevalence of Traumatic Encephalopathy among Ex-Professional Boxers.* London: Pitman Medical and Scientific Publishing.

Roberts, G. W., D. Allsop, and C. Bruton. 1990. "The Occult Aftermath of Boxing." *Journal of Neurology Neurosurgery and Psychiatry* 53(5): 373–378.

Roberts, G. W., H. L. Whitwell, P. R. Acland, et al. 1990. "Dementia in a Punch-Drunk Wife." *Lancet* 335(8694):918–919.

Roberts, G. W., S. M. Gentleman, A. Lynch, et al. 1991. "βA4 Amyloid Protein Deposition in Brain after Head Trauma." *Lancet* 338: 1422–1423.

Schwarz, A. 2007. "Expert Ties Ex-Player's Suicide to Brain Damage." *New York Times,* January 18.

Smith, D. H., V. E. Johnson, and W. Stewart. 2013. "Chronic Neuropathologies of Single and Repetitive TBI: Substrates of Dementia?" *Nature Reviews: Neurology* 9:211–221.

Stern, R. A., D. H. Daneshvar, C. M. Baugh, et al. 2013. "Clinical Presentation of Chronic Traumatic Encephalopathy." *Neurology* 81: 1122–1129.

Sullan, M. J., B. M. Asken, and M. S. Jaffee. 2018. "Glymphatic System Disruption as a Mediator of Brain Trauma and Chronic Traumatic Encephalopathy." *Neuroscience and Biobehavioral Reviews* 84:316–324.

Tagge, C. A., A. M. Fisher, O. V. Minaeva, et al. 2018. "Concussion, Microvascular Injury, and Early Tauopathy in Young Athletes after Impact Head Injury and an Impact Concussion Mouse Model." *Brain* 141(2):422–458.

Washington, P. M., S. Villapol, and M. P. Burns. 2016. "Polypathology and Dementia after Brain Trauma: Does Brain Injury Trigger Distinct Neurodegenerative Diseases or Should They Be Classified Together as Traumatic Encephalopathy?" *Experimental Neurology* 275:381–388.

Weir, D. R., J. S. Jackson, and A. Sonnega. 2009. "National Football League Player Care Foundation: Study of Retired NFL Players." Institute for Social Research, University of Michigan, Ann Arbor. http://ns.umich.edu/Releases/2009/Sep09/FinalReport.pdf.

Chapter 5 • Exercising Sensibly

American Association of Neurological Surgeons. n.d. "Sports–Related Head Injury." https://www.aans.org/en/Patients/Neurosurgical-Conditions -and-Treatments/Sports-related-Head-Injury. Accessed May 27, 2019.

Anderson, M. 2014. "Bike Use Is Rising among the Young, but It Is Sky-rocketing among the Old." People for Bikes, Boulder, CO, June 19. https://peopleforbikes.org/blog/bike-use-is-rising-among-the-young-but-it-is-skyrocketing-among-the-old/.

Benham, E. C., S. W. Ross, M. Mavilia, et al. 2017. "Injuries from All-Terrain Vehicles: An Opportunity for Injury Prevention." *American Journal of Surgery* 214(2):211–216.

Benson, B. W., G. M. Hamilton, W. H. Meeuwisse, et al. 2009. "Is Pro-tective Equipment Useful in Preventing Concussion? A Systematic Review of the Literature." *British Journal of Sports Medicine* 43(suppl. 1):i56–i67.

Bombeck, E. 1985/1996. *Four of a Kind: A Suburban Field Guide.* Bbs Publishing.

Boniface, K., M. P. McKay, R. Lucas, et al. 2011. "Serious Injuries Related to the Segway® Personal Transporter: A Case Series." *Annals of Emer-gency Medicine* 57(4):370–374.

Burke, M. 2018. "Olympic Bobsledder Raises Concussion Awareness." Concussion Legacy Foundation, Boston, January 28. https://concussion foundation.org/story/olympic-bobsledder-raises-concussion-aware ness.

Butts, C. C., J. W. Rostas, Y. L. Lee, et al. 2015. "Larger ATV Engine Size Correlates with an Increased Rate of Traumatic Brain Injury." *Injury* 46(4):625–628.

Carmichael, S. P., D. L. Davenport, P. A. Kearney, et al. 2014. "On and Off the Horse: Mechanisms and Patterns of Injury in Mounted and Unmounted Equestrians." *Injury* 45(9):1479–1483.

Cheng, T. A., J. M. Bell, T. Haileyesus, et al. 2016. "Nonfatal Playground-Related Traumatic Brain Injuries among Children, 2001–2013." *Pedi-atrics* 137(6):e20152721.

Cuenca, A. G., A. Wiggins, M. K. Chen, et al. 2009. "Equestrian Injuries in Children." *Journal of Pediatric Surgery* 44(1):148–150.

Denning, G. M., and C. A. Jennissen. 2016. "What You May Not Know about All-Terrain Vehicle-Related Deaths and Injuries." *Annals of Emergency Medicine* 68(3):396–397.

FIS Surveillance System: 2006–2018. 2018. Oslo Sports Trauma Research Center, May. https://assets.fis-ski.com/image/upload/v1537433416/fis-prod/assets/FIS_ISS_report_2017-18_English.pdf.

Goel, V., and Q. Hardy. 2015. "Dave Goldberg, Silicon Valley Executive, Died of Head Trauma, Mexican Official Says." *New York Times,* May 4.

Jefferson, T. Letter to John Garland Jefferson, 1790.

Kasmire, K. E., S. C. Rogers, and J. J. Sturm. 2016. "Trampoline Park and Home Trampoline Injuries." *Pediatrics* 138(3):e20161236.

Laver, L., I. P. Pengas, and O. Mei-Dan. 2017. "Injuries in Extreme Sports." *Journal of Orthopaedic Surgery and Research* 12(1):59.

Linnaus, M. E., R. L. Ragar, E. M. Garvey, et al. 2017. "Injuries and Outcomes Associated with Recreational Vehicle Accidents in Pediatric Trauma." *Journal of Pediatric Surgery* 52(2):327–333.

Loder, R. T., and S. Abrams. 2011. "Temporal Variation in Childhood Injury from Common Recreational Activities." *Injury* 42(9):945–957.

Mohn, T. 2018. "The Dutch Reach: A No-Tech Way to Save Bicyclists' Lives." *New York Times,* October 5.

National Ski Areas Association. Lids on Kids Program. http://www.nsaa.org/safety-programs/lids-on-kids/. Accessed May 27, 2019.

Safe Kids Worldwide. 2016. Bicycle, Skate, and Skateboard Safety Fact Sheet. https://www.safekids.org/fact-sheet/bicycle-skate-and-skateboard-safety-fact-sheet-2016-pdf.

Sanford, T., C. E. McCulloch, R. A. Callcut, et al. 2015. "Bicycle Trauma Injuries and Hospital Admissions in the United States, 1998–2013." *JAMA* 314(9):947–949.

Siracuse, B. L., J. A. Ippolito, P. D. Gibson, et al. 2017. "Hoverboards: A New Cause of Pediatric Morbidity." *Injury* 48(6):1110–1114.

Sone, J. Y., D. Kondziolka, J. H. Huang, et al. 2017. "Helmet Efficacy against Concussion and Traumatic Brain Injury: A Review." *Journal of Neurosurgery* 126(3):768–781.

Srinivasan, V., C. Pierre, B. Plog, et al. 2014. "Straight from the Horse's Mouth: Neurological Injury in Equestrian Sports." *Neurological Research* 36(10):873–877.

Trivedi, T. K., C. Liu, A. L. M. Antonio, et al. 2019. "Injuries Associated with Standing Scooter Use." *JAMA Network: Open* 2(1) e187381.

Tuakli-Wosorno, Y., and W. Derman, eds. 2018. "Para and Adapted Sports Medicine." *Physical Medicine and Rehabilitation Clinics of North America* 29(2):185–426.

Twain, M. 1917 / 1992. "Taming the Bicycle." In *Mark Twain: Collected Tales, Sketches, Speeches, and Essays 1852–1890,* ed. Louis J. Budd. New York: Library of America. https://loa-shared.s3.amazonaws.com/static/pdf/Twain_Taming_Bicycle.pdf. See p. 89.

Villegas, C. V., S. M. Bowman, C. K. Zogg, et al. 2016. "The Hazards of Off-Road Motor Sports: Are Four Wheels Better Than Two?" *Injury* 47(1):178–183.

Webborn, N., C. A. Blauwet, W. Derman, et al. 2017. "Heads Up on Concussion in Para Sport." *British Journal of Sports Medicine* 52(18):1157–1158.

Winkler, E., J. K. Yuh, J. F. Burke, et al. 2016. "Adult Sports-Related Traumatic Brain Injury in United States Trauma Centers." *Neurosurgical Focus* 40(4):E4.

Zuckerman, S. L., C. D. Morgan, S. Burks, et al. 2015. "Functional and Structural Traumatic Brain Injury in Equestrian Sports: A Review of the Literature." *World Neurosurgery* 83(6):1098–1113.

Chapter 6 • Game Changers

Alosco, M. L., A. B. Kasimis, J. M. Stamm, et al. 2017. "Age of First Exposure to American Football and Long-Term Neuropsychiatric and Cognitive Outcomes." *Translational Psychiatry* 7(9):e1236.

American Academy of Pediatrics Council on Sports Medicine and Fitness. 2015. "Tackling in Youth Football." *Pediatrics* 136(5):e1419.

Bachynski, K. 2016. "Tolerable Risks? Physicians and Youth Tackle Football." *New England Journal of Medicine* 374(5):405–407.

Baugh, C., E. Kroshus, D. H. Daneshvar, et al. 2014. "Concussion Management in United States College Sports: Compliance with National Collegiate Athletic Association Policy and Areas for Improvement." *American Journal of Sports Medicine* 43(1):47–56.

Baugh, K., and Z. E. Shapiro. 2015. "Concussions and Youth Football: Using a Public Health Law Framework to Head Off a Potential Public Health Crisis." *Journal of Law and the Biosciences* 2(2):449–458.

Belson, K. 2016. "Pop Warner Settles Lawsuit over Player Who Had CTE." *New York Times,* March 9.

Benson, B. W., A. S. McIntosh, D. Maddocks, et al. 2013. "What Are the Most Effective Risk-Reduction Strategies in Sport Concussion?" *British Journal of Sports Medicine* 47(5):321–326.

Bieler, D. 2017. "North Carolina Bill Would Have Allowed Parents of Concussed Kids to Authorize Return to Play." *Washington Post,* February 28.

Boden, B. P., R. L. Tacchetti, R. C. Cantu, et al. 2007. "Catastrophic Head Injuries in High School and College Football Players." *American Journal of Sports Medicine* 35(7):1075–1081.

Brenner, J. S. 2016. "Sports Specialization and Intensive Training in Young Athletes." *Pediatrics* 138(3):e20162148.

Cantu, R. C., and J. K. Register-Mihalik. 2011. "Considerations for Return-to-Play and Retirement Decisions after Concussion." *PM&R* 3(10):S440–S444. See p. S441.

Carson, J. D., D. W. Lawrence, S. A. Kraft, et al. 2014. "Premature Return to Play and Return to Learn after a Sport-Related Concussion: Physician's Chart Review." *Canadian Family Physician* 60(6):e310–315.

Centers for Disease Control and Prevention. 2015. "Sports Prevention Policies and Laws: Information for Parents, Coaches, and School and Sports Professionals." https://www.cdc.gov/headsup/policy/index.html.

Colvin, A. C., J. Mullen, M. R. Lovell, et al. 2009. "The Role of Concussion History and Gender in Recovery from Soccer-Related Concussion." *American Journal of Sports Medicine* 37(9):1699–1704.

Comstock, R. D., D. W. Currie, L. A. Pierpoint, et al. 2015. "An Evidence-Based Discussion of Heading the Ball and Concussions in High School Soccer." *JAMA Pediatrics* 169(9):830–837.

Davis-Hayes, C., D. R. Baker, T. S. Bottiglieri, et al. 2018. "Medical Retirement from Sport after Concussions: A Practical Guide." *Neurology: Clinical Practice* 8(1):40–47.

Dollé, J.-P., A. Jaye, S. A. Anderson, et al. 2018. "Newfound Sex Differences in Axonal Structure Underlie Differential Outcomes from in Vitro Traumatic Axonal Injury." *Experimental Neurology* 300:121–134.

Dompier, T. P., Z. Y. Kerr, S. W. Marshall, et al. "Incidence of Concussion during Practice and Games in Youth, High School, and Collegiate American Football Players." *JAMA Pediatrics* 169(7):659–665.

Ekstrand, J., T. Timpka, and M. Hägglund. 2006. "Risk of Injury in Elite Football Played on Artificial Turf versus Natural Grass: A Prospective Two-Cohort Study." *British Journal of Sports Medicine* 40(12):975–980.

Elbin, R. J., A. Sufrinko, P. Schatz, et al. 2016. "Removal from Play after Concussion and Recovery Time." *Pediatrics* 138(3):e20160910.

Emery, C. A., A. M. Black, A. Kolstad, et al. 2018. "What Strategies Can Be Used to Effectively Reduce the Risk of Concussion in Sport? A Systematic Review." *British Journal of Sports Medicine* 51:978–984.

Gallant, F., J. L. O'Loughlin, J. Brunet, et al. 2017. "Childhood Sports Participation and Adolescent Sport Profile." *Pediatrics* 140(6):e20171449.

Graham, R., F. P. Rivera, M. A. Ford, et al., eds. 2014. *Sports Related Concussions in Youth: Improving the Science, Changing the Culture.* Washington, DC: Institute of Medicine and the National Research Council of the National Academies, National Academies Press. See p. 7.

Kerr, Z. Y., S. L. Dalton, K. G. Roos, et al. 2016. "Comparison of Indiana High School Football Injury Rates by Inclusion of the USA Football 'Heads Up Football' Player Safety Coach." *Orthopaedic Journal of Sports Medicine* 4(5):2325967116648441.

Kerr, Z. Y., R. Hayden, T. P. Dompier, et al. 2015. "Association of Equipment Worn and Concussion Injury Rates in National Collegiate Athletic Association Football Practices: 2004–2005 to 2008–2009 Academic Years." *American Journal of Sports Medicine* 43(5):1134–1141.

Kerr, Z. Y., S. W. Yeargin, T. C. V. McLeod, et al. 2015. "Comprehensive Coach Education Reduces Head Impact Exposure in American Youth Football." *Orthopedic Journal of Sports Medicine* 3(10):1–6.

Kroshus, E., B. Garnett, M. Hawrilenko, et al. 2015. "Concussion Under-Reporting and Pressure from Coaches, Teammates, Fans, and Parents." *Social Science & Medicine* 134:66–75.

Kroshus, E., Z. Y. Kerr, and J. G. L. Lee. 2017. "Community-Level Inequities in Concussion Education of Youth Football Coaches." *American Journal of Preventive Medicine* 52(4):476–482.

Laker, S. R., A. Meron, M. R. Greher, et al. 2016. "Retirement and Activity Restrictions Following Concussion." *Physical Medicine and Rehabilitation Clinics of North America* 27(2):487–501.

Lawrence, D. W., P. Comper, M. G. Hutchinson, et al. 2016. "Influence of Extrinsic Risk Factors on National Football League Injury Rates." *Orthopaedic Journal of Sports Medicine* 4(3):2325967116639222.

Lynall, R. C., T. C. Mauntel, D. A. Padua, et al. 2015. "Acute Lower Extremity Injury Rates Increase after Concussion in College Athletes." *Medicine and Science in Sports and Exercise* 47(12):2487–2492.

Mandela, N. 2000. Acceptance Speech: Laureus World Sports Awards Ceremony, Monaco, France, May 25.

McCrory, P., W. Meeuwisse, J. Dvorak, et al. 2017. "Consensus Statement on Concussion in Sport: The 5th International Conference on Concussion in Sport Held in Berlin, October 2016." *British Journal of Sports Medicine* 51(11):838–847.

McLendon, L. A., S. F. Kralik, P. A. Grayson, et al. 2016. "The Controversial Second Impact Syndrome: A Review of the Literature." *Pediatric Neurology* 62:9–17.

Myer, G. D., W. Yuan, K. D. B. Foss, et al. 2016. "Analysis of Head Impact Exposure and Brain Microstructure Response in a Season-Long Application of a Jugular Vein Compression Collar: A Prospective, Neuroimaging Investigation in American Football." *British Journal of Sports Medicine* 50(20):1276–1285.

Nanos, K. N., J. M. Franco, D. Larson, et al. 2017. "Youth Sport-Related Concussions: Perceived and Measured Baseline Knowledge of Concussions among Community Coaches, Athletes, and Parents." *Mayo Clinic Proceedings* 92(12):1782–1790.

Nordström, A., P. Nordström, and J. Ekstrand. 2014. "Sports-Related Concussion Increases the Risk of Subsequent Injury by about 50% in Elite Male Football Players." *British Journal of Sports Medicine* 19:1447–1450.

O'Connor, K. L., S. Rowson, S. M. Duma, et al. 2017. "Head-Impact–Measurement Devices: A Systematic Review." *Journal of Athletic Training* 52(3):206–227.

Omalu, B. 2015. "Don't Let Kids Play Football." Op-ed, *New York Times,* December 17, A23.

Patel, D. R., D. Fidrocki, and V. Parachuri. 2017. "Sport-Related Concussions in Adolescent Athletes: A Critical Public Health Problem for Which Prevention Remains an Elusive Goal." *Translational Pediatrics* 6(3):114–120.

Ransom, D. M., C. G. Vaughan, L. Pratson, et al. 2015. "Academic Effects of Concussion in Children and Adolescents." *Pediatrics* 135(6):1043–1050.

Reynolds, B. B., J. Patrie, E. J. Henry, et al. 2016. "Practice Type Effects on Head Impact in Collegiate Football." *Journal of Neurosurgery* 124(2):501–510.

Rowson, S., R. W. Daniel, and S. M. Duma. 2013. "Biomechanical Performance of Leather and Modern Football Helmets." *Journal of Neurosurgery* 119(3):805–809.

Sarmiento, K., Z. Donnell, and R. Hoffman. 2017. "A Scoping Review to Address the Culture of Concussion in Youth and High School Sports." *Journal of School Health* 87(10):790–804.

Schmidt, J. D., K. Rizzone, N. L. Hoffman, et al. 2018. "Age at First Concussions Influences the Number of Subsequent Concussions." *Pediatric Neurology* 81:19–34.

Smith, D. H., V. E. Johnson, and W. Stewart. 2013. "Chronic Neuropathologies of Single and Repetitive TBI: Substrates of Dementia?" *Nature Reviews: Neurology* 9:211–221. See p. 212.

Smoliga, J., and G. W. Zavorsky. 2017. "'Tighter Fit' Theory—Physiologists Explain Why 'Higher Altitude' and Jugular Occlusion Are Unlikely to Reduce Risks for Sports Concussion and Brain Injuries." *Journal of Applied Physiology* 122:215–217.

Stamm, J. M., A. P. Bourlas, C. M. Baugh, et al. 2015. "Age of First Exposure to Football and Later-Life Cognitive Impairment in Former NFL Players." *Neurology* 84(11):1114–1120.

Stamm, J. M., I. K. Koerte, M. Muehlmann, et al. 2015. "Age of First Exposure to Football Is Associated with Altered Corpus Callosum White Matter Microstructure in Former Professional Football Players." *Journal of Neurotrauma* 32:1768–1776.

Stemper, B. D., A. S. Shah, J. Hareziak, et al. 2018. "Comparison of Head Impact Exposure between Concussed Football Athletes and Matched Controls: Evidence for a Possible Second Mechanism of Sport-Related Concussion." *Annals of Biomedical Engineering,* online October 22.

Swartz, E. E., S. P. Broglio, S. B. Cook, et al. 2015. "Early Results of a Helmetless-Tackling Intervention to Decrease Head Impacts in Football Players." *Journal of Athletic Training* 50(12):1219–1222.

Underwood, J. 1979. *Death of an American Game.* New York: Harper-Collins.

Vrentas, J. 2017. "The Quest for a Better Football Helmet." *Sports Illustrated,* May 31. https://www.si.com/mmqb/2017/05/31/nfl-quest-better -football-helmet.

Wallace, J., T. Covassin, and E. Beidler. 2017. "Sex Differences in High School Athletes' Knowledge of Sport-Related Concussion Symptoms and Reporting Behaviors." *Journal of Athletic Training* 52(7):682–688.

Wallace, J., T. Covassin, S. Nogle, et al. 2017. "Knowledge of Concussion and Reporting Behaviors in High School Athletes with or without Access to an Athletic Trainer." *Journal of Athletic Training* 52(3):228–235.

Waltzman, D., and K. Sarmiento. 2019. "What the Research Literature Says about the Risk Factors and Prevention Strategies for Youth Sports: A Scoping Review of Six Commonly Played Sports." *Journal of Safety Research* 68:157–172.

Wasserman, E. B., J. J. Bazarian, M. Mapstone, et al. 2016. "Academic Dysfunction after a Concussion among US High School and College Students." *American Journal of Public Health* 106(7):1247–1253.

Wiebe, D. J., B. A. D'Alonzo, R. Harris, et al. 2018. "Association between the Experimental Kickoff Rule and Concussion Rates in Ivy League Football." *JAMA* 320(19):2035–2036.

Zambito, T. 2013. "Family of Football Player Ryne Dougherty Who Died in 2008 Settles Lawsuit for 2.8 Million." *NJ.com,* September 10. https://www.nj.com/essex/index.ssf/2013/09/family_of_montclair _high_school_football_player_ryne_dougherty_who_died_in_2008 _settles_lawsuit_for.html

Zemper, E. D. 2003. "Two-Year Prospective Study of Relative Risk of a Second Cerebral Concussion." *American Journal of Physical Medicine and Rehabilitation* 82(9):653–659.

Zuckerman, S. L, Z. Y. Kerr, A. Yengo-Kahn, et al. 2015. "Epidemiology of Sports-Related Concussion in NCAA Athletes from 2009–2010 to 2013–2014: Incidence, Recurrence, and Mechanisms." *American Journal of Sports Medicine* 43(11):2654–2663.

Chapter 7 ▪ Money Talks

"5th Annual Super Bowl Survey Highlights." 2018. Burson-Marsteller, January 26. https://www.slideshare.net/Burson-Marsteller/5th-annual-super-bowl-survey.

Bachynski, K., and D. S. Goldberg. 2018. "Time Out: NFL Conflicts of Interest with Public Health Efforts to Prevent TBI." *Injury Prevention* 24(3):180–184.

Badenhausen, K. 2017. "How Roger Goodell's $200 Million Payday Compares to America's Top CEOs." *Forbes,* December 7.

———. 2019. "The Average Player Salary and Highest-Pain in NBA, MLB, NHL, NFL and MLS." *Forbes,* May 27.

Belson, K. 2014. "Brain Trauma to Affect One in Three Players, NFL Agrees." *New York Times,* September 12.

———. 2017. "Team Relocations Keep NFL Moving Up Financially." *New York Times,* January 12.

———. 2018. "Football's True Believers Circle the Wagons and Insist the Sport Is Just Fine." *New York Times,* January 30.

Belson, K., and A. Schwarz. 2016. "NFL Shifts on Concussion and Game May Never Be the Same." *New York Times,* March 15.

Cohen, I. G., H. F. Lynch, and C. R. Deubert. 2016. "A Proposal to Address NFL Club Doctors' Conflicts of Interest and to Promote Player Trust." *Hastings Center Special Report,* November / December, S2–S24.

Deubert, C. R., I. G. Cohen, and H. F. Lynch. 2016. "Protecting and Promoting the Health of NFL Players: Legal and Ethical Analysis and Recommendations." The Petrie-Flom Center for Health Law Policy, Biotechnology, and Bioethics at Harvard Law School, Cambridge,

MA. https://petrieflom.law.harvard.edu/resources/article/new-report -protecting-and-promoting-the-health-of-nfl-players.

Drape, J. 2018. "The Youth Sports Megacomplex Comes to Town Hoping Teams Will Follow." *New York Times,* September 12.

Fair, R. C., and C. Champa. 2018. "Estimated Costs of Contact in High School Male Sports." *Journal of Sports Economics* 20(5):690–717.

Fairanu, S., and M. Fairanu-Wada. 2016. "Congressional Report Says NFL Waged Improper Campaign to Influence Government Study." ESPN .com. May 22, updated May 24. http://www.espn.com/espn/otl/story /_/id/15667689/congressional-report-finds-nfl-improperly -intervened-brain-research-cost-taxpayers-16-million.

Gaul, G. M. 2015. *Billion-Dollar Ball: The Big Money Culture of College Football.* New York: Viking.

"Global Sports Salaries Survey." 2018. *Sporting Intelligence.* https:// globalsportssalaries.com.

Gregory, S. 2017. "How Kid Sports Turned Pro." *Time* 190(9), September 4.

Holland, K., and J. W. Schoen. 2014. "Think Athletic Scholarships Are a 'Holy Grail'? Think Again." CNBC, October 13. https://www.cnbc .com/2014/10/13/think-athletic-scholarships-are-a-holy-grail-think -again.html.

Kang, C. 2014. "How the Government Helps the NFL Maintain Its Power and Profitability." *Washington Post,* September 16.

Kirk, J. 2014. "25 Maps That Explain College Football." *SB Nation* sports blog, August 20. https://www.sbnation.com/college-football/2014/8 /20/6030683/25-maps-that-explain-college-football.

Kirschen, M. P., A. Tsou, and S. B. Nelson. 2014. "Legal and Ethical Implications in the Evaluation and Management of Sports–Related Concussion." *Neurology* 83(4):352–358. See p. 355.

Lavigne, P. 2016. "Rich Get Richer in College Sports as Poor Schools Struggle to Keep Up." ESPN.com, September 2. https://abcnews.go

.com/Sports/rich-richer-college-sports-poorer-schools-struggle /story?id=41857422.

Leibovich, M. 2018. *Big Game: The NFL in Dangerous Times*. New York: Penguin.

Leopold, S. S., M. B. Dobbs, M. C. Debhart, et al. 2016. "Editorial: Do Orthopaedic Surgeons Belong on the Sidelines of American Football Games." *Journal of Orthopaedics and Related Research* 475:2615–2617. See p. 2617.

Lundberg, G. D. 1983. "Boxing Should Be Banned in Civilized Countries." *JAMA* 249(2):250.

———. 2016. "The NFL's Collision with the Future." *New York Times,* February 4, A27.

McCrory, P., W. Meeuwisse, J. Dvorak, et al. 2017. "Consensus Statement on Concussion in Sport: The 5th International Conference on Concussion in Sport Held in Berlin, October 2016." *British Journal of Sports Medicine* 51(11):838–847. See p. 847.

National Football League. 2016. "Statement on Congressional Committee NIH Report." *NFL.com,* May 23.http://www.nfl.com/news/story /oap3000000664453/article/nfl-statement-on-congressional -committee-nih-report.

Norman, J. 2018. "Football Still Americans' Favorite Sport to Watch." Gallup, January 4. https://news.gallup.com/poll/224864/football -americans-favorite-sport-watch.aspx.

Patterson, T. 2018. "America's Incredibly Expensive Football Stadiums." CNN, September 28. https://www.cnn.com/2018/09/28/us/expensive -college-football-stadiums/index.html.

PWC Sports Outlook. 2018. "At the Gate and Beyond: Outlook for the Sports Market in North America through 2021." https://www.pwc .com/us/en/industries/tmt/library/sports-outlook-north-america .html.

Roberts, J. L., I. G. Cohen, C. R. Deubert, et al. 2017. "Evaluating NFL Player Health and Performance: Legal and Ethical Issues." *University of Pennsylvania Law Review* 165(2):227–314.

Schwarz, A. 2016. "NFL-Backed Youth Program Says It Reduced Concussions: The Data Disagrees." *New York Times,* July 27.

Sirota, D. 2013. "The Sports-Industrial Complex Is Bleeding America Dry." Salon.com, February 8.https://www.salon.com/2013/02/08/the _sports_industrial_complex_is_bleeding_america_dry/.

Smith, C. 2018. "College Football's Most Valuable Teams: Texas A&M Jumps to Number 1." *Forbes,* September 11.

Strauss, B. 2016. "Six Concussion Lawsuits Are Filed against Colleges and the NCAA." *New York Times,* May 16.

Tagliabue, P. 2017. "Tagliabue Exclusive: My 1994 Concussion Remarks 'A Mistake.'" Interview with Clark Judge, Talk of Fame Network, February 1. http://www.talkoffamenetwork.com/tagliabue-exclusive -1994-concussions-remars-mistae/.

Union of Concerned Scientists. "The Disinformation Playbook: How Business Interests Deceive, Misinform, and Buy Influence at the Expense of Public Safety." https://www.ucsusa.org/our-work/center-science-and -democracy/disinformation-playbook#.W_h2d5NKhYM. Accessed May 27, 2019.

WinterGreen Research, Inc. 2018. "Youth Team, League, and Tournament Sports: Market Shares, Strategies, and Forecasts, Worldwide, 2018 to 2024." Press release, September 1. http://www.wintergreenresearch .com/youth-sports.

Chapter 8 • Close to Home

Bergen, G., M. R. Stevens, and E. R. Burns. 2016. "Falls and Fall Injuries among Adults Aged ≥65 Years—United States, 2014." *MMWR Morbidity and Mortality Weekly Report* 65(37):993–998.

Campbell, J. C., J. C. Anderson, A. McFadgion, et al. 2018. "The Effects of Intimate Partner Violence and Probable Traumatic Brain Injury on

Central Nervous System Symptoms." *Journal of Women's Health* 27(6):761–767.

Centers for Disease Control and Prevention (CDC). 2011. "Traumatic Brain Injury in Prisons and Jails: An Unrecognized Problem." http://www.cdc.gov/traumaticbraininjury/pdf/Prisoner_TBI_Prof-a .pdf.

———. 2017. "Important Facts about Falls." https://www.cdc.gov /homeandrecreationalsafety/falls/adultfalls.html.

Choudhary, A. K., S. Servaes, T. L. Slovis, et al. 2018. "Consensus Statement on Abusive Head Trauma in Infants and Young Children." *Pediatric Radiology* 48(8):1048–1065.

Christensen, J., M. G. Pedersen, C. B. Pedersen, et al. 2009. "Long-Term Risk of Epilepsy after Traumatic Brain Injury in Children and Young Adults: A Population-Based Cohort Study." *Lancet* 373(9669): 1105–1110.

Coats, B., and S. S. Margulies. 2008. "Potential for Head Injuries in Infants from Low-Height Falls." *Journal of Neurosurgery and Pediatrics* 2(5):321–330.

Colantonio, A., H. Kim, S. Allen, et al. 2014. "Traumatic Brain Injury and Early Life Experiences among Men and Women in a Prison Population." *Journal of Correctional Health Care* 20(4):271–279.

Corrigan, J. D., M. Wolfe, W. J. Mysiw, et al. 2003. "Early Identification of Mild Traumatic Brain Injury in Female Victims of Domestic Violence." *American Journal of Obstetrics and Gynecology* 188(5 suppl.): S71–S76.

Crowe, L., A. Collie, S. Hearps, et al. 2016. "Cognitive and Physical Symptoms of Concussive Injury in Children: A Detailed Longitudinal Recovery Study." *British Journal of Sports Medicine* 50(5):311–316.

Dams-O'Connor, K., L. E. Gibbons, J. D. Bowen, et al. 2013. "Risk for Late-Life Re-Injury, Dementia and Death among Individuals with Traumatic Brain Injury: A Population-Based Study." *Journal of Neurology, Neurosurgery and Psychiatry* 84(2):177–182.

Davis, A. 2014. "Violence-Related Mild Traumatic Brain Injury in Women: Identifying a Triad of Postinjury Disorders." *Journal of Trauma Nursing* 21(6):300–308.

Dichter, M. E., C. Cerulli, and R. M. Bossarte. 2011. "Intimate Partner Violence Victimization among Women Veterans and Associated Heart Health Risks." *Women's Health Issues* 21(4 suppl.):S190–S194.

Durand, E., M. Chevignard, A. Ruet, et al. 2017. "History of Traumatic Brain Injury in Prison Populations: A Systematic Review." *Annals of Physical and Rehabilitation Medicine* 60:95–101.

Farrer, T. J., and D. W. Hedges. 2011. "Prevalence of Traumatic Brain Injury in Incarcerated Groups Compared to the General Population: A Meta-Analysis." *Progress in Neuro-Psychopharmacology and Biological Psychiatry* 35(2):390–394.

Fazel, S., P. Lichtenstein, M. Grann, et al. 2011. "Risk of Violent Crime in Individuals with Epilepsy and Traumatic Brain Injury: A 35-Year Swedish Population Study." *PLoS Med* 8:e1001150.

Fazel, S., A. Wolf, D. Pillas, et al. 2014. "Suicide, Fatal Injuries, and Other Causes of Premature Mortality in Patients with Traumatic Brain Injury a 41-Year Swedish Population Study." *JAMA Psychiatry* 71(3):326–333.

Gaist, D., L. A. G. Rodriguez, M. Hellfritzsch, et al. 2017. "Association of Antithrombotic Drug Use with Subdural Hematoma Risk." *JAMA* 317(8):836–846.

Gardner, R. C., K. Dams-O'Connor, M. R. Morrissey, et al. 2017. "Geriatric Traumatic Brain Injury: Epidemiology, Outcomes, Knowledge Gaps, and Future Directions." *Journal of Neurotrauma* 35: 889–906.

Gaw, C. E., T. Chounthirath, G. A. Smith, et al. 2016. "Nursery Product-Related Injuries Treated in United States Emergency Departments." *Pediatrics* 139(4):e20162503.

Geddes, J. F., A. K. Hackshaw, G. H. Vowles, et al. 2001. "Neuropathology of Inflicted Head Injury in Children. I. Patterns of Brain Damage." *Brain* 124:1290–1298.

Geddes, J. F., G. H. Vowles, A. K. Hackshaw, et al. 2001. "Neuropathology of Inflicted Head Injury in Children II. Microscopic Brain Injury in Infants." *Brain* 124:1299–1306.

Goldin, Y., H. L. Haag, and C. T. Trott. 2016. "Screening for History of Traumatic Brain Injury among Women Exposed to Intimate Partner Violence." *PM&R* 8(11):1104–1110.

Graupman, P., and K. R. Winston. 2006. "Nonaccidental Head Trauma as a Cause of Childhood Death." *Journal of Neurosurgery: Pediatrics* 104(4):245–250.

Hinds, T., E. Shalaby-Rana, A. M. Jackson, et al. 2015. "Aspects of Abuse: Abusive Head Trauma." *Current Problems in Pediatric and Adolescent Health Care* 45(3):71–79.

Iverson, K. M., and T. K. Pagoda. 2015. "Traumatic Brain Injury among Women Veterans: An Invisible Wound of Intimate Partner Violence." *Medical Care* 53:S112–S119.

Iverson, K. M., N. A. Sayer, M. Meterko, et al. 2017. "Intimate Partner Violence among Female OEF/OIF/OND Veterans Who Were Evaluated for Traumatic Brain Injury in the Veterans Health Administration: A Preliminary Investigation." *Journal of Interpersonal Violence,* 1–24. doi:10.1177/0886260517702491.

Iverson, K. M., S. W. Stirman, A. E. Street, et al. 2016. "Female Veterans' Preferences for Counseling Related to Intimate Partner Violence: Informing Patient-Centered Interventions." *General Hospital Psychiatry* 40:33–38.

Kaba, F., P. Diamond, A. Haque, et al. 2014. "Traumatic Brain Injury among Newly Admitted Adolescents in the New York City Jail System." *Journal of Adolescent Health* 54(5):615–617.

Karakurt, G., V. Patel, K. Whiting, et al. 2017. "Mining Electronic Health Records Data: Domestic Violence and Adverse Health Effects." *Journal of Family Violence* 32(1):79–87.

Kwako, L. E., N. Glass, J. Campbell, et al. 2011. "Traumatic Brain Injury in Intimate Partner Violence: A Critical Review of Outcomes and Mechanisms." *Trauma Violence and Abuse* 12:115–126.

Lachs, M. S., and K. A. Pillemer. 2015. "Elder Abuse." *New England Journal of Medicine.* 373(20):1947–1956.

Lafferty, B. 2010. "Traumatic Brain Injury: A Factor in the Causal Pathway to Homelessness?" *Journal for Nurse Practitioners* 6(5):358–362.

Lind, K., H. Toure, D. Brugel, et al. 2016. "Extended Follow-up of Neurological, Cognitive, Behavioral and Academic Outcomes after Severe Abusive Head Trauma." *Child Abuse and Neglect* 51: 358–367.

Lindberg, D. M., B. Beaty, E. Juarez-Colunga, et al. 2015. "Testing for Abuse in Children with Sentinel Injuries." *Pediatrics* 136(5):831–838.

McIsaac, K. E., A. Moser, R. Moineddin, et al. 2016. "Association between Traumatic Brain Injury and Incarceration: A Population-Based Cohort Study." *Canadian Medical Association Journal* 4(4): e746–e753.

McKinlay, A., R. Grace, J. Horwood, et al. 2009. "Adolescent Psychiatric Symptoms Following Preschool Childhood Mild Traumatic Brain Injury: Evidence from a Birth Cohort." *Journal of Head Trauma Rehabilitation* 24(3):221–227.

Mian, M., J. Shah, A. Dalpiaz, et al. 2015. "Shaken Baby Syndrome: A Review." *Fetal and Pediatric Pathology* 34(3):169–175.

Miller, E., and B. McCaw. 2019. "Intimate Partner Violence." *New England Journal of Medicine* 380:850–857.

Miller, T. R., R. Steinbeigle, A. Wicks, et al. 2014. "Disability-Adjusted Life-Year Burden of Abusive Head Trauma at Ages 0–4." *Pediatrics* 134(6):e1545–e1550.

Nadarasa, J., C. Deck, F. Meyer, et al. 2014. "Update on Injury Mechanisms in Abusive Head Trauma–Shaken Baby Syndrome." *Pediatric Radiology* 44(Suppl 4):S565–S570.

Piccolino, A. L., and K. B. Solberg. 2014. "The Impact of Traumatic Brain Injury on Prison Health Services and Offender Management." *Journal of Correctional Health* 20(3):203–212.

Sariaslan, A., D. J. Sharp, B. M. D'Onofrio, et al. 2016. "Long-Term Outcomes Associated with Traumatic Brain Injury in Childhood and Adolescence: A Nationwide Swedish Cohort Study of a Wide Range of Medical and Social Outcomes." *PLoS Med* 13(8):e1002103.

Schofield, P. W., E. Malacova, D. B. Preen, et al. 2015. "Does Traumatic Brain Injury Lead to Criminality? A Whole-Population Retrospective Cohort Study Using Linked Data." *PLoS One* 10(7):e0132558.

Shapiro, F. 2018. *Eye Movement Desensitization and Reprocessing [EMDR] Therapy: Basic Principles, Protocols, and Procedures,* 3rd edition. New York: Guilford Press.

Shiroma, E. J., P. L. Ferguson, and E. E. Pickelsimer. 2010. "Prevalence of Traumatic Brain Injury in an Offender Population: A Meta-Analysis." *Journal of Correctional Health Care* 16(2):147–159.

Simonnet, H., A. Laurent-Vannier, W. Yuan, et al. 2014. "Parents' Behavior in Response to Infant Crying: Abusive Head Trauma Education." *Child Abuse and Neglect* 38(12):1914–1922.

St. Ivany, A., L. Bullock, D. Shminkey, et al. 2018. "Living in Fear and Prioritizing Safety: Exploring Women's Lives after Traumatic Brain Injury from Intimate Partner Violence." *Qualitative Health Research* 11:1708–1718.

St. Ivany, A., and D. Schminkey. 2016. "Intimate Partner Violence and Traumatic Brain Injury: State of the Science and Next Steps." *Family and Community Health* 39(2):129–137.

Stevens, J. A., and E. A. Phalen. 2013. "Development of STEADI: A Fall Prevention Resource for Health Care Providers." *Health Promotion and Practice* 14(5):706–714.

Svoboda, T., and J. T. Ramsay. 2014. "High Rates of Head Injury among Homeless and Low Income Housed Men: A Retrospective Cohort Study." *Emergency Medicine Journal* 31(7):571–575.

Topolovec-Vranic, J., A. Schuler, A. Gozdzik, et al. 2017. "The High Burden of Traumatic Brain Injury and Comorbidities amongst Homeless Adults with Mental Illness." *Journal of Psychiatric Research* 87:53–60.

Trachtenberg, F. L., E. A. Haas, H. C. Kinney, et al. 2012. "Risk Factor Changes for Sudden Infant Death Syndrome after Initiation of Back-to-Sleep Campaign." *Pediatrics* 129:630–638.

United States Department of Health and Human Services, Children's Bureau. 2016. "Child Maltreatment 2016." https://www.acf.hhs.gov/sites/default/files/cb/cm2016.pdf.

Valera, E. M., A. Cao, O. Pasternak, et al. 2019. "White Matter Correlates of Mild Traumatic Brain Injury in Women Subjected to Intimate-Partner Violence: A Preliminary Study." *Journal of Neurotrauma* 36(5): 661–668.

Voelker, R. 2018. "For Survivors of Intimate Partner Violence, Overlooked Brain Injuries Take a Toll." *Medical News and Perspectives: JAMA* 320(6):535–537.

Wennberg, R., C. Hiploylee, P. Tai, et al. 2018. "Is Concussion a Risk Factor for Epilepsy?" *Canadian Journal of Neurological Sciences* 45: 275–282.

Whitehead, A. N. 1925. *Science and the Modern World*. Lowell Lectures. New York: Macmillan. See p. 207.

Williams, W. H., P. Chitsabesan, S. Fazel, et al. 2018. "Traumatic Brain Injury: A Potential Cause of Violent Crime?" *Lancet Psychiatry* 5(10):836–844. See p. 838.

Wong, J. Y-H, D. Y-T. Fong, V. Lai, et al. 2014. "Bridging Intimate Partner Violence and the Human Brain." *Trauma, Violence, and Abuse* 15(1):22–33.

Wright, J. N. 2017. "CNS Injuries in Abusive Head Trauma." *American Journal of Roentgenology* 208(5):991–1001.

Chapter 9 ▪ War and Work

Adam, O., C. L. MacDonald, D. Rivet, et al. 2015. "Clinical and Imaging Assessment of Acute Combat Mild Traumatic Brain Injury in Afghanistan." *Neurology* 85(3):219–227.

Agoston, D., P. Arun, P. Bellgowan, et al. 2017. "Military Blast Injury and Chronic Neurodegeneration: Research Presentations from the 2015 International State-of-the-Science Meeting." *Journal of Neurotrauma* 34(S1):S6–S17.

American Psychiatric Association. 1980. *Diagnostic and Statistical Manual of Mental Disorders (DSM-III)*, 3rd edition. Arlington, VA: American Psychiatric Association.

Bailie, J. M., J. E. Kennedy, L. M. French, et al. 2016. "Profile Analysis of the Neurobehavioral and Psychiatric Symptoms Following Combat-Related Mild Traumatic Brain Injury: Identification of Subtypes." *Journal of Head Trauma Rehabilitation* 31(1):2–12.

Barnes, D. E., A. Kaup, K. Kirby, et al. 2014. Traumatic Brain Injury and Risk of Dementia in Older Veterans." *Neurology* 83(4):312–319.

Baxter, D., D. J. Sharp, C. Feeney, et al. 2013. "Pituitary Dysfunction after Blast Traumatic Brain Injury: The UK BIOSAP Study." *Annals of Neurology* 74(4):527–536.

Belanger, H. G., T. Kretzmer, R. D. Vanderploeg, et al. 2010. "Symptom Complaints Following Combat-Related Traumatic Brain Injury: Relationship to Traumatic Brain Injury Severity and Posttraumatic Stress Disorder." *Journal of the International Neuropsychological Society* 16(1):194–199.

Benge, J. F., N. J. Pastorek, and G. M. Thornton. 2009. "Postconcussive Symptoms in OEF-OIF Veterans: Factor Structure and Impact of Posttraumatic Stress." *Rehabilitation Psychology* 54(3):270–278.

Bryant, R. A. 2008. "Disentangling Mild Brain Injury and Stress Reaction." *New England Journal of Medicine* 358(5):525–527. See p. 526.

Bureau of Labor Statistics. 2018. "2017 Census of Fatal Occupational Injuries Charts." https://www.bls.gov/iif/oshwc/cfoi/cfch0016.pdf

Capehart, B., and D. Bass. 2012. "Review: Managing Posttraumatic Stress Disorder in Combat Veterans with Comorbid Traumatic Brain Injury." *Journal of Rehabilitation Research and Development* 49(5):789–812.

Casper, S. T. 2014. *The Neurologists: A History of a Medical Specialty in Modern Britain, c. 1789–2000.* Manchester, UK: Manchester University Press.

Centers for Disease Control and Prevention. "The National Institute for Occupational Safety and Health (NIOSH)." https://www.cdc.gov /niosh/index.htm. Accessed September 17, 2019.

Cifu, D., B. Taylor, W. F. Carne, et al. 2013. "Traumatic Brain Injury, Post-Traumatic Stress Disorder, and Pain Diagnoses in OIF / OEF / OND Veterans." *Journal of Rehabilitation, Research and Development* 50(9): 1169–1176.

Cifu, D., S. I. Cohen, H. L. Lew, et al. 2010. "History and Evolution of Traumatic Brain Injury Rehabilitation in Military Service Members and Veterans." *American Journal of Physical Medicine and Rehabilitation* 89(8):688–694.

Defense and Veterans Brain Injury Center. https://dvbic.dcoe.mil/. Accessed September 17, 2019.

de Koning, M. E., M. E. Myrthe, H. D. van der Horn, et al. 2017. "Prediction of Work Resumption and Sustainability up to 1 Year after Mild Traumatic Brain Injury." *Neurology* 89(18):1908–1914.

DePalma, R. G., and S. W. Hoffman. 2018. "Combat Blast Related Traumatic Brain Injury (TBI): Decade of Recognition; Promise of Progress." *Behavioural Brain Research* 340:102–105.

Ferdosi, H., K. A. Schwab, A. Metti, et al. 2018. "Trajectory of Post-Concussive Symptoms 12-Months Post-Deployment in Soldiers with and without Mild Brain Injury—Warrior STRONG Study." *American Journal of Epidemiology* 188(1):77–86.

Fazel, S., A. Wolf, D. Pillas, et al. 2014. "Suicide, Fatal Injuries, and Other Causes of Premature Mortality in Patients with Traumatic Brain Injury: A 41-Year Swedish Population Study." *JAMA Psychiatry* 71(3): 326–333.

Fralick, M., E. Sy, and A. Hassan. 2019. "Association of the Risk of Suicide with Concussion." *JAMA Neurology* 76(2):144–151.

Garber, B. G., C. Rusu, M. A. Zamorski, et al. 2016. "Occupational Outcomes Following Mild Traumatic Brain Injury in Canadian Military Personnel Deployed in Support of the Mission in Afghanistan: A Retrospective Cohort Study." *BMJ Open* 6(5):e010780.

Greer, N., N. Sayer, M. Kramer, et al. 2016. "Prevalence and Epidemiology of Combat Blast Injuries from the Military Cohort 2001–2014." VA ESP Project #09-009.

Grinker, R. R., and J. P. Spiegel. 1943. *War Neuroses in North Africa: The Tunisian Campaign.* New York: The Josiah Macy, Jr. Foundation. See p. 139.

Hayes, J. P., D. R. Miller, G. Lafleche, et al. 2015. "The Nature of White Matter Abnormalities in Blast-Related Mild Traumatic Brain Injury." *Neuroimage: Clinical* 8:148–156.

Hillenbrand, L. 2001. *Seabiscuit: An American Legend.* New York: Random House. See p. 77.

Hitchens, P. L., A. E. Hill, and S. M. Stover. 2013. "Jockey Falls, Injuries, and Fatalities Associated with Thoroughbred and Quarter-Horse Racing in California, 2007–2011." *Orthopedic Journal of Sports Medicine.* doi: 10.1177/2325967113492625.

Hoge, C. W., H. M. Goldberg, and C. A. Castro. 2009. "Care of War Veterans with Mild Traumatic Brain Injury—Flawed Perspectives." *New England Journal of Medicine* 360(16):1588–1593.

Hoge, C. W., D. McGerk, J. L. Thomas, et al. 2008. "Mild Traumatic Brain Injury in Soldiers Returning from Iraq." *New England Journal of Medicine* 358(5):453–463.

Holtkamp, M. D., J. Grimes, and G. Ling. 2016. "Concussion in the Military: An Evidence-Base Review of MTBI in US Military Personnel Focused on Posttraumatic Headache." *Current Pain and Headache Reports* 20:37.

Johnson, D. 2017. "The Top 10 Most Dangerous Jobs in America." *Time,* December 27, 8–9.

Jones, E. 2010. "Shell Shock at Maghull and the Maudsley: Models of Psychological Medicine in the UK." *Journal of the History of Medicine and the Allied Health Sciences* 65(3):368–395.

———. 2014. "'An Atmosphere of Cure': Frederick Mott, Shell Shock and the Maudsley." *History of Psychiatry* 25(4):412–421.

Jones, E., N. T. Fear, and W. Wessely, "Shell Shock and Mild Traumatic Brain Injury: A Historical Review." *American Journal of Psychiatry* 164:1641–1645.

Kaufman, H. H. 1993. "Treatment of Head Injuries in the American Civil War." *Journal of Neurosurgery* 78(5):838–845.

Konda, S. "Traumatic Brain Injuries in Construction." 2016. National Institute for Occupational Safety and Health (NIOSH) Science Blog, Centers for Disease Control and Prevention, March 21. https://blogs.cdc.gov/niosh-science-blog/2016/03/21/constructiontbi/.

Konda, S., A. Reichard, H. M. Tiesman, et al. 2015. "Non-Fatal Work-Related Traumatic Brain Injuries Treated in US Hospital Emergency Departments, 1998–2007." *Injury Prevention* 21(2):115–120.

Lange, R. T., T. A. Brickell, J. E. Kennedy, et al. 2014. "Factors Influencing Postconcussion and Posttraumatic Stress Symptom Reporting Following Military-Related Concurrent Polytrauma and Traumatic Brain Injury." *Archives of Clinical Neuropsychology* 29(4):329–347.

MacDonald, C. L., J. Barber, M. Jordan, et al. 2017. "Early Clinical Predictors of 5-Year Outcome after Concussive Blast Traumatic Brain Injury." *JAMA Neurology* 74(7):821–829.

Magnuson, J., F. Leonessa, and G. S. F. Ling. 2012. "Neuropathology of Explosive Blast Traumatic Brain Injury." *Current Neurology and Neuroscience Reports* 12(5):570–579.

Matérne, M., L-O. Lundqvist, and T. Strandberg. 2017. "Opportunities and Barriers for Successful Return to Work after Acquired Brain Injury: A Patient Perspective." *Work* 56(1):125–134.

McDonald, M. C., M. Brandt, and R. Bluhm. 2017. "From Shell-Shock to PTSD, a Century of Invisible War Trauma." *The Conversation,* April 3. https://theconversation.com/from-shell-shock-to-ptsd-a-century-of-invisible-war-trauma-74911.

McKee, A. C., and M. E. Robinson. 2014. "Military-Related Traumatic Brain Injury and Neurodegeneration." *Alzheimer's and Dementia* 10(3 suppl.):S242–S253.

Mott, F. W. 1917. "The Microscopic Examination of the Brains of Two Men Dead of Commotio Cerebri (Shell Shock) without Visible External Injury." *British Medical Journal* 2(2967):612.

Mu, W., E. Catenaccio, and M. L. Lipton. 2017. "Neuroimaging in Blast-Related Mild Traumatic Brain Injury." *Journal of Head Trauma Rehabilitation* 32(1):55–69.

Nordlöf, H., B. Wiitavaara, H. Högberg, et al. 2017. "A Cross-Sectional Study of Factors Influencing Occupational Health and Safety Management Practices in Companies." *Safety Science* 95:92–103.

Omalu, B., J. L. Hammers, and J. Bailes. 2011. "Chronic Traumatic Encephalopathy in an Iraqi War Veteran with Posttraumatic Stress Disorder Who Committed Suicide." *Neurosurgical Focus* 31(5):E3.

Ownsworth, T., and K. McKenna. 2004. "Investigation of Factors Related to Employment Outcome Following Traumatic Brain Injury a Critical

Review and Conceptual Model." *Disability and Rehabilitation* 26(13): 765–784.

Park, E., R. Eisen, A. Kinio, et al. 2013. "Electrophysiological White Matter Dysfunction and Association with Neurobehavioral Deficits Low-Level Primary Blast Trauma." *Neurobiology of Disease* 52:150–159.

Press, J. M., Davis, D. D., S. L. Wiesner, et al. 1995. "The National Jockey Injury Study: An Analysis of Injuries to Professional Horse-Racing Jockeys." *Clinical Journal of Sport Medicine* 5:236–240.

Raji, C. A., K. Willeumier, D. Taylor, et al. 2015. "Functional Neuroimaging with Default Mode Network Regions Distinguishes PTSD from TBI in a Military Veteran Population." *Brain Imaging and Behavior* 9(3):527–534.

Ramati, A., N. H. Pliskin, S. Keedy, et al. 2009. "Alteration in Functional Brain Systems after Electrical Injury." *Journal of Neurotrauma* 26:1815–1822.

Riedy, G., J. S. Senseney, W. Liu, et al. 2016. "Findings from Structural MR Imaging in Military Traumatic Brain Injury." *Radiology* 279(1):207–215.

Rigg, J. L., and S. R. Mooney. 2011. "Concussions and the Military: Issues Specific to Service Members." *PM&R* 3(10 suppl. 2):S380–S386.

Rosenfeld, J. V, A. C. McFarlane, P. Bragge, et al. 2013. "Blast-Related Traumatic Brain Injury." *Lancet Neurology* 12(9):882–893.

Russell, J. A., and B. M. Daniell. 2018. "Concussion in Theatre: A Cross-Sectional Survey of Prevalence and Management in Actors and Theater Technicians." *Journal of Occupational and Environmental Medicine* 60(3):205–210.

Shively, S. B., and D. P. Perl. 2017. "Viewing the Invisible Wound: Novel Lesions Identified in Postmortem Brains of US Service Members with Military Blast Exposure." *Military Medicine* 182(1):1461–1463.

Shively, S. B., I. Horkayne-Szakaly, R. V. Jones, et al. 2016. "Characterisation of Interface Astroglial Scarring in Human Brain after Blast Exposure: A Post-Mortem Case Series." *Lancet Neurology* 15:944–953.

Silverberg, N. D., W. J. Panenka, and G. L. Iverson. 2018. "Work Productivity Loss after Mild Traumatic Brain Injury." *Archives of Physical Medicine and Rehabilitation* 99(2):250–256.

Steinhauer, J. 2019. "V. A. Officials, and the Nation, Battle an Unrelenting Tide of Veteran Suicides." *New York Times,* April 14.

Suri, P., K. Stolzmann, K. M. Iverson, et al. 2017. "Associations between Traumatic Brain Injury History and Future Headache Severity in Veterans: A Longitudinal Study." *Archives of Physical Medicine and Rehabilitation* 98(11):2118–2125.

Tanielian, T., and L. H. Jaycox, eds. 2008. *Invisible Wounds of War: Psychological and Cognitive Injuries, Their Consequences, and Services to Assist Recovery.* Santa Monica, CA: RAND.

Terry, D. P., G. L. Iverson, W. Panenka, et al. 2018. "Workplace and Non-Workplace Mild Traumatic Brain Injuries in an Outpatient Clinic Sample: A Case-Control Study." *PLoS One* 13(6):1–17.

Theadom, A., S. Barker-Collo, K. Jones, et al. 2017. "Work Limitations 4 Years after Mild Traumatic Brain Injury: A Cohort Study." *Archives of Physical Medicine and Rehabilitation* 98(8):1560–1566.

Undurti, A., E. A. Colasurdo, C. L. Sikkema, et al. 2018. "Chronic Hypopituitarism Associated with Postconcussive Symptoms Is Prevalent after Blast-Induced Mild Brain Injury." *Frontiers of Neurology* 9:72.

United States Department of Labor. Occupational Safety and Health Administration. "How to File a Safety and Health Complaint." https://www.osha.gov/workers/file_complaint.html. Accessed September 14, 2019.

van der Molen, H. F., P. Basnet, P. L. T. Hoonakker, et al. 2018. "Interventions to Prevent Injuries in Construction Workers." *Cochrane Database of Systematic Reviews* 2018(2):9–11.

Vincent, A. S., T. M. Roebuck-Spencer, and A. Cernich. 2014. "Cognitive Changes and Dementia Risk after Traumatic Brain Injury: Implications for Aging Military Personnel." *Alzheimer's and Dementia* 10(3 suppl.): S174–S187.

Walilko, T., C. North, L. A. Young, et al. 2009. "Head Injury as a PTSD Predictor among Oklahoma Bombing Survivors." *Journal of Trauma* 67(6):1311–1319.

Wall, S. E., W. H. Williams, S. Cartwright-Hatton, et al. 2006. "Neuro-psychological Dysfunction Following Repeat Concussions in Jockeys." *Journal of Neurology, Neurosurgery and Psychiatry* 77(4):518–520.

Xu, L., M. L. Schaefer, R. M. Linville, et al. 2016. "Neuroinflammation in Primary Blast Neurotrauma: Time Course and Prevention by Torso Shielding." *Experimental Neurology* 277:268–274.

Yaffe, K., E. Vittinghoff, K. Lindquist, et al. 2010. "Posttraumatic Stress Disorder and Risk of Dementia among US Veterans." *Archives of General Psychiatry* 67(6):608–613.

Yeh, P-H., C. Guan Koay, B. Wang, et al. 2017. "Compromised Neurocir-cuitry in Chronic Blast-Related Mild Traumatic Brain Injury." *Human Brain Mapping* 38:352–369.

Conclusion

Caro, D. H. J. 2011. "Traumatic Brain Injury Care Systems: 2020 Trans-formational Challenges." *Global Journal of Health Science* 3(1):19–29.

Maas, A. I. R., D. K. Menon, H. F. Lingsma, et al. 2012. "Re-orientation of Clinical Research in Traumatic Brain Injury: Report of an Interna-tional Workshop on Comparative Effectiveness Research." *Journal of Neurotrauma* 29:32–46.

Maas, A. R., D. K. Menon, and P. D. Adelson. 2017. "Traumatic Brain Injury: Integrated Approaches to Improve Prevention, Clinical Care, and Research in Traumatic Brain Injury: A Global Challenge." *Lancet* 16(12): 987–1048.

Manley, G., and A. Maas. 2013. "Traumatic Brain Injury: An International Knowledge-Based Approach." *JAMA* 310(5):473–474.

Roozenbeek, B., A. I. R. Maas, and D. K. Menon. 2013. "Changing Patterns in the Epidemiology of Traumatic Brain Injury." *Nature Review, Neurology* 9:231–236.

Tosetti, P., R. R. Hicks, E. Theriault et al. 2013. "Toward an International Initiative for Traumatic Brain Injury Research." *Journal of Neurotrauma* 30:1211–1222.

Wilson, L., W. Stewart, K. Dams-O'Connor, et al. 2017. "The Chronic and Evolving Neurological Consequences of Traumatic Brain Injury." *Lancet* 16:813–825.

ACKNOWLEDGMENTS

MANY PEOPLE HELPED to make this book possible. I owe huge debts to my mentors at the Medical College of Pennsylvania (now Drexel College of Medicine), Jefferson Medical School (now the Sidney Kimmel School of Medicine), Thomas Jefferson University Hospital, and Magee Rehabilitation Hospital for teaching me neuroscience and humanistic approaches in the practice of medicine. My primary fellowship supervisor, physiatrist Lawrence Horn, and other fellowship mentors—neurologist Sanford Auerbach, and physiatrists Mel Glenn and the late Sheldon Berrol—taught me brain injury medicine.

Many colleagues have influenced my thinking, as have so many patients and their families. While working in trauma systems, rehabilitation hospitals, and practice settings in Pennsylvania, New Jersey, and California, I had opportunities to learn from them about care and care delivery for people with traumatic injuries. At the University of Pennsylvania, I gained experience from colleagues in neuroimaging research. I learned about population-based research from colleagues at the Northern California Kaiser Permanente Division of Research. My other colleagues in the Kaiser Permanente health-care system, and especially at Kaiser Foundation Rehabilitation Center and Hospital in Vallejo, California, enabled me to learn about providing care to people within an integrated health system.

I thank my expert and dedicated colleagues at Paradigm, based in Walnut Creek, California, who support high-quality care for injured workers and their families, and the Department of Physical Medicine and Rehabilitation at the University of California, Davis, where I have been able to teach and learn with academic colleagues and residents.

Fellow physiatrist and colleague Julie Silver jumpstarted me in the early stages of book writing through the Harvard University writing course for health-care professionals that she directs. My agent, Jeanne Fredericks, provided me with key guidance and support. None of my efforts would have been possible without my skilled editor, Janice Audet, and her team at Harvard University Press.

My deep appreciation goes to the expert reviewers who volunteered their precious time to read manuscript drafts and whose comments strengthened the book: physiatrists David Cifu, Maya Evans, Mel Glenn, Melita Moore, Steven Moskowitz, and Nathan Zasler; neuropsychologists Ernest Bryant and Iris Weber; neurosurgeon Andrew Maas; neuro-optometrist Jacqueline Theis; emergency medicine physician Michael Choo; anesthesiologist Seth Fischer; medical historian Stephen Casper; economist Elyce Rotella; epidemiologist Sarah Ackley; internist Brigid McCaw; sports aficionado Paul Epstein, my brother-in-law; coach Joe Fama; and medical society executive Thomas Stautzenbach.

My writing group gave me kind yet incisive critiques and kept me on track: Abbe Blum, Julia Epstein, Rena Fraden, Gayle Green, Carol Joffe, Catherine Kudlick, Jeanne Marechek, Randy Milden, and Judith Newton. Medical historian Janet Golden guided me on book publishing and provided a crucial introduction to Stephen Casper.

Robert Wayne Woods was a wonderful collaborator who masterfully created all of the book's illustrations. Marilyn Anderson created the comprehensive index.

I received well-informed advice for my website (www.elizabethsandelmd .com) and social media activities from Rusty Shelton and the Advantage Media Group and from Click Cape Cod. The following people volunteered their time for video interviews or other content for the website: Cheri Blauwet, Ernest Bryant, Michelle Camicia, Anthony Chen, Richard Delmonico, Maya Evans, Seth Fischer, Steven Flanagan, Kam Gardiner, Mel Glenn, Hetal Lakhani, James McDeavitt, Maureen Miner, Melita Moore, Steven Moskowitz, Michael O'Dell, Richard Reyes, Raymond Samatovicz, Beverly Swann, and Jacqueline Theis. My morning walking group in Oakland helped me counter the many hours of sitting with my computer and offered pertinent advice and resources: Julia Epstein, Jerry Jacobs, Lois Jacobs, Susan Lindheim, Jim Spencer, Pajes Sterman, and Kaki and Tib Tusler.

The one person to whom I owe my world, including this book, is my spouse and best friend, Julia Epstein. She is my anchor and my best advisor for all things literary. Our daughters, Anna and Maria, son-in-law, Max, and grandson, Gio, keep our lives interesting and fulfilling as their stories unfold. Gio is almost always a glass half full and persistently curious. At age 2, while I was in the final stages of writing this book, his two favorite questions were "What doing?" and "Why?" These are, in fact, two fundamental questions for all of us as we attempt to make sense of, and hopefully change for the better, the world in which we live. This book is my contribution to those efforts.

INDEX

Note: Page numbers in *italics* indicate illustrations.